AF833410

NEUROBLASTOMA - CURRENT STATE AND RECENT UPDATES

Edited by **Chandrika Gowda**

Neuroblastoma - Current State and Recent Updates
http://dx.doi.org/10.5772/66615
Edited by Chandrika Gowda

Contributors

Evelyne Ségal-Bendirdjian, Joëlle El Hajj, Delphine Garsuault, Claire Bouyer, Eric Nguyen, George Hilal, Çığır Biray Avcı, Bakiye Goker Bagca, Tamer Hasan Hassan, Francesca F Caputi, Sanzio Candeletti, Patrizia Romualdi, Sandrine Valsesia-Wittmann, Tala Shekarian, Gian Paolo Tonini, Murat Tosun, Hamit Selim Karabekir, Nuket Gocmen Mas, Yasemin Soysal, Harun Muayad Muayad Said, Mehmet Ozan Durmaz, Neema Bhat, Lisa McGregor

Published by InTech
Janeza Trdine 9, 51000 Rijeka, Croatia

© The Editor(s) and the Author(s) 2017
The moral rights of the editor(s) and the author(s) have been asserted.
All rights to the book as a whole are reserved by InTech. The book as a whole (compilation) cannot be reproduced, distributed or used for commercial or non-commercial purposes without InTech's written permission. Enquiries concerning the use of the book should be directed to InTech's rights and permissions department (permissions@intechopen.com).
Violations are liable to prosecution under the governing Copyright Law.

Individual chapters of this publication are distributed under the terms of the Creative Commons Attribution 3.0 Unported License which permits commercial use, distribution and reproduction of the individual chapters, provided the original author(s) and source publication are appropriately acknowledged. More details and guidelines concerning content reuse and adaptation can be found at http://www.intechopen.com/copyright-policy.html.

Notice

Statements and opinions expressed in the chapters are these of the individual contributors and not necessarily those of the editors or publisher. No responsibility is accepted for the accuracy of information contained in the published chapters. The publisher assumes no responsibility for any damage or injury to persons or property arising out of the use of any materials, instructions, methods or ideas contained in the book.

Publishing Process Manager Maja Bozicevic
Technical Editor SPi Global
Cover InTech Design team

First published October, 2017
Printed in Croatia
Legal deposit, Croatia: National and University Library in Zagreb

Additional hard copies can be obtained from orders@intechopen.com

Neuroblastoma - Current State and Recent Updates , Edited by Chandrika Gowda
p. cm.
Print ISBN 978-953-51-3583-8
Online ISBN 978-953-51-3584-5

We are IntechOpen, the world's leading publisher of Open Access books

Built by scientists, for scientists

3,500+
Open access books available

111,000+
International authors and editors

115M+
Downloads

151
Countries delivered to

Our authors are among the
Top 1%
most cited scientists

12.2%
Contributors from top 500 universities

CLARIVATE ANALYTICS BOOK CITATION INDEX INDEXED

WEB OF SCIENCE™

Selection of our books indexed in the Book Citation Index in Web of Science™ Core Collection (BKCI)

Interested in publishing with us?
Contact book.department@intechopen.com

Numbers displayed above are based on latest data collected.
For more information visit www.intechopen.com

For EU product safety concerns:
IN TECH d.o.o., Prolaz Marije Krucifikse Kozulić 3, 51000 Rijeka, Croatia,
info@intechopen.com or visit our website at intechopen.com.

Meet the editor

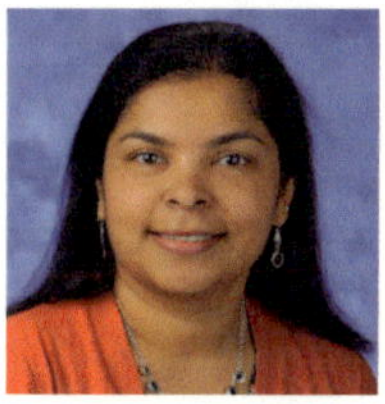

Dr. Chandrika Gowda received her medical training in India. She went on to complete her residency training in Pediatrics at the Unterberg Children's Hospital at Monmouth Medical Center, New Jersey, and fellowship training in Hematology-Oncology at the Penn State Children's Hospital in Hershey, Pennsylvania. Dr. Gowda is currently a board certified Pediatric Hematologist-Oncologist and has served as an Assistant Professor of pediatrics at Pennsylvania State University College of Medicine for the past 4 years. Dr. Gowda is a physician scientist with major efforts committed toward conducting basic science and translation research in addition to treating children with various cancers. Her research is focused on targeting oncogenic signaling pathways and designing novel targeted therapies in order to treat pediatric cancers like leukemia and neuroblastoma. The main focus of her research is to understand the function of Ikaros tumor suppressor and the regulation of Ikaros activity in childhood cancers, including leukemia and neuroblastoma. She has published several research articles, reviews, and book chapters to her credit. She has also presented her work at various national and international scientific platforms and gained national recognition for her work.

Contents

Preface

Neuroblastoma (NBL) is a unique embryonal tumor that arises from neural crest cells. These cells form the sympathetic nervous system and are present as mass in various locations in the body. It is also unique in terms of tumor biology and natural outcome of the disease in various age groups. A newborn with NBL has the greatest chance of spontaneous regression, whereas an older child is more likely to have high-risk metastatic disease at diagnosis with poor prognosis. Neuroblastoma is the most common extracranial solid tumor of childhood, with about 700 new cases of neuroblastoma seen each year in the United States. The 5-year survival rate for children with high-risk NBL is only 50–60%, and this survival rate has not improved over the last 10 years. A child diagnosed with high-risk NBL has the best chance of remission when treated with a multimodality treatment approach that includes chemotherapy, surgical excision, radiotherapy, myeloablative chemotherapy followed by stem cell rescue, immunotherapy, and use of biological agents, among others. This book is a compilation of various chapters intended to provide basic knowledge to readers about the clinical presentation, staging, current standard of treatment, and various newer treatment strategies that are forthcoming. Given the poor outcomes for a specific subgroup of patients with high-risk disease, it is not surprising that this field has attracted hundreds of researchers over several decades who have dedicated their work to better understanding the genetics and biology of this tumor type and who are keen to design novel targeted therapies. Each subspecialist (medical oncologist, radiation oncologist, and surgeon) involved in a child's treatment has expertise in certain aspects of the treatment, and thus the first several chapters here are focused on providing a concise overview that will be useful for all providers involved in the treatment of patients with neuroblastoma.

There have been many advances in the treatment of neuroblastoma in recent years including therapeutic MIBG, immunotherapy, and personalized targeted therapy based on the genetic alterations seen in tumor. The primary objective of this book is to provide the readers with a comprehensive review of neuroblastoma—clinical aspects and the currently available treatment along with the recent advancements and future directions in the field of NBL treatment. The topics and chapters have been compiled keeping in mind a diverse group of readers in different areas of specialty such as pediatric oncology, surgery, radiation oncology, and immunology, as well as physician scientists and basic researchers working in the field of neuroblastoma.

Chandrika Gowda, MD
Assistant Professor of Pediatrics, Hematology-Oncology
Penn State Health Medical Center
Pennsylvania State University College of Medicine,
Hershey, Pennsylvania, USA

Chapter 1

Neuroblastoma: The Clinical Aspects

Neema Bhat and Lisa McGregor

Additional information is available at the end of the chapter

http://dx.doi.org/10.5772/intechopen.70486

Abstract

Neuroblastoma is a predominantly pediatric cancer, arising from the primordial neural crest cells that form the sympathetic nervous system. The prognosis for patients with neuroblastoma can vary from uniform survival in low risk patients to fatality in patients with high risk disease. This chapter gives a brief overview of the epidemiology, genetics, clinical presentation, diagnosis, and discussion of the various staging systems and risk classifications of neuroblastoma. We also briefly describe our understanding of the conventional and novel treatment modalities available and their effects on the current prognosis of patients with neuroblastoma. The purpose of this chapter is to serve as a brief overview of the clinical aspects of neuroblastoma, to serve as a foundation of knowledge for scientists aspiring to develop new therapeutic modalities for this dreadful pediatric disease.

Keywords: neuroblastoma, epidemiology, clinical presentation, diagnosis, clinical staging and risk stratification, prognosis, current treatment modalities, novel and targeted therapy

1. Introduction

Neuroblastoma is a neoplasm arising from the primordial neural crest cells that form the sympathetic nervous system. It is a cancer predominantly seen in pediatric patients. It is the most common extracranial malignancy of childhood and the most common solid tumor of infancy [1]. It is one of the most enigmatic tumors with extremely heterogeneous clinical behavior that ranges from spontaneous regression to metastatic disease refractory to therapy. It accounts for about 7% of all childhood malignancies; however 10% of childhood cancer related mortality. Treatment approaches have been based on presence or absence of specific clinical or biologic factors. Although substantial progress has been made in the treatment and outcomes for low and intermediate risk neuroblastoma, success in therapy of high risk neuroblastoma remains

INTECH
open science | open minds

© 2017 The Author(s). Licensee InTech. This chapter is distributed under the terms of the Creative Commons Attribution License (http://creativecommons.org/licenses/by/3.0), which permits unrestricted use, distribution, and reproduction in any medium, provided the original work is properly cited.

evasive and complicated. Patients with low and intermediate risk neuroblastoma have an overall survival rate exceeding 90% and are now moving toward minimization of therapy [2]. However in spite of standard therapy for high risk neuroblastoma patients involving multi-agent chemotherapy induction, surgery and external beam radiotherapy, myeloablative chemotherapy with autologous hematopoietic stem cell rescue and biologic agents, only 50% of patients with newly diagnosed high risk disease will survive [2].

1.1. Origin and embryology

The neural crest is an embryonic structure formed at the beginning of the 4th week of human development. These cells migrate to the trunk to form the sympathetic ganglia and adrenal medulla, however little is known about the molecular events governing the formation and migration of these cells.

However it is important to note that although Neuroblastoma tumors can have neural crest cell traits, they also share properties of extra-adrenal chromaffin cells as reviewed in [3].

1.2. Epidemiology

The incidence of neuroblastoma is 10.5 per million children between 0 and 14 years of age in North America and Europe. There is a slight male preponderance of 1.2:1.0 [1]. The median age of diagnosis for neuroblastoma in patients is 19 months (ranging from 0 to 4 years). In fact one study reported that 16% of infant neuroblastomas were diagnosed during the 1st month of life (i.e. neonatal) and 41% during the first 3 months [4]. Less than 5% of neuroblastomas are diagnosed at 10 years of age or older [5]. Although there are no significant geographic variations in the incidence, African American and Native American patients are more likely to have high risk disease features and poor outcomes due to genetic differences [6].

1.3. Genetics

Genetics form a major part of risk stratification, targeted treatment and prognosis markers for neuroblastoma. Although *MYCN* amplification was found as early as in 1983, the finding of further genes involved in oncogenesis took much longer [7]. However, over the past decade this has changed significantly, due to the advances made in exome and whole-genome sequencing [7]. In addition to *MYCN*, two other oncogenes, *ALK* [8] and *LIN28B* [9] were also found to be amplified, although in much lower frequency.

1.4. Oncodriver genes in neuroblastoma

1.4.1. MYCN

Karyotyping on neuroblastoma was frequently found to reveal gene amplifications. The *MYC* related oncogene *MYCN* (2p24) was originally identified by Schwab and colleagues [10, 11] as a target of this amplification event. It was later found that amplification of MYCN is associated with advanced stages of disease, unfavorable biologic features and poor prognosis [12, 13].

It was also found to be independently associated with poor outcome in otherwise favorable patient groups [14, 15]. At present, the *MYCN* gene status is determined routinely at diagnosis for therapy planning. Fluorescent in situ hybridization is the preferred technique for detection of *MYCN* amplification. Most groups define amplification as >4 times the number of MYCN copies as compared to a control probe. In most tumors with MYCN amplification, the copy number is often as high as 50–400 copies/cell. MYCN amplification has been found to be a mutation present at diagnosis and not one that is acquired with tumor progression. MYCN is a member of the proto-oncogene family and is responsible for expression of approximately 15% of all human genes. Hence overexpression causes a significant impact on cell behaviors.

1.4.2. ALK

The developing nervous system has been found to express a cell surface receptor tyrosine kinase controlled by the ALK (Anaplastic Lymphoma Kinase) gene [16]. Germline ALK mutations are the major cause of hereditary neuroblastoma as described below, however somatically acquired ALK-activating mutations are also found as oncogenic drivers in 8–10% of sporadic neuroblastoma [16]. In combination with tumors that also exhibit MYCN amplification, 10–14% of neuroblastoma tumors have an ALK alteration that may serve as a novel therapeutic target. Crizotinib (one of the first ALK inhibitors) is currently being tested in neuroblastoma [17].

1.5. Hereditary predisposition to neuroblastoma and associated syndromes

The incidence of familial neuroblastoma is estimated to be 1–2% [1]. It is very unusual for an individual neuroblastoma patient to have a family history positive for neuroblastoma [18]. Analysis of rare family pedigree charts, are strongly supportive of an autosomal dominant inheritance with incomplete penetrance [8, 19]. Familial disease has the same diverse clinical behavior as sporadic neuroblastoma, ranging from aggressive progression to spontaneous regression. Genetic cases most often are seen to have multifocal and/or bilateral adrenal primary tumors. The median age of onset for familial neuroblastoma is at around 9 months of age. Familial neuroblastoma patients differ from their sporadic counterparts in that they are diagnosed at an earlier age and/or with multiple primary tumors and are associated with other cancer predisposition syndromes [20–22].

Missense, nonsense and polyalanine repeat expansion mutations in PHOX2B were collectively found to be responsible for approximately 5% of hereditary neuroblastomas [23]. PHOX2B is a homeobox gene and is a key regulator of normal autonomic nervous system development and inactivating mutations of this gene account for this rare field defect of sympathoadrenal tissues.

Detailed studies involving familial pedigrees identified germ line mutations in the tyrosine kinase domain of the Anaplastic Lymphoma Kinase (*ALK*) oncogene [24]. Sporadic neuroblastoma tumors also can harbor ALK abnormalities in about 8–12% cases. Hence, collectively, gain of function mutations in ALK or inactivating mutations of PHOX2B account for 80–85% of hereditary neuroblastomas. Therefore genetic testing for mutations in these two genes should be strongly considered in a patient who has a family history of neuroblastoma or has evidence of multiple primary tumors like bilateral adrenal tumors. If these mutations are found, these patients should be followed by appropriate genetic counseling and should be closely monitored as per cancer surveillance protocols. However there are still 15–20% of hereditary neuroblastoma cases still unaccounted for by these mutations, making it likely that one or more additional predisposition genes perhaps remain to be discovered.

From literature and multiple case reviews and review of family pedigree charts, it is now known that neuroblastoma can occur in other neural crest disorders (like Hirschsprung disease, Central Hypoventilation Syndrome and Neurofibromatosis NF1) [20]. These conditions have been given the collective term Neurocristopathy syndromes and can have difference therapeutic implications.

In addition to the Neurocristopathy syndromes, NB cases are also seen in other familial cancer syndromes like Beckwith-Weidemann syndrome (art2ref38), Noonan syndrome, Li-Fraumeni syndrome [25, 26], Fanconi anemia and other chromosomal breakage syndromes [21, 27].

2. Clinical presentation

Clinical presentation in patients with neuroblastoma varies based on the primary tumor locations which may occur anywhere along the sympathetic chain and on the extent of disease. The clinical presentation can be varied and is a combination of symptoms from the primary tumor and metastatic disease.

2.1. Localized disease

Most of the primary tumors arise in the abdomen (75%) of which a vast majority of them involve the adrenal gland. Frequency of adrenal tumors in older children is higher (40%) compared to infants (25%), infants tend to have more cervical and thoracic tumors [18].

Patients with primary adrenal tumors may have a varying range of symptoms from being asymptomatic or can be associated with hypertension, abdominal pain, distension and constipation. Sudden hemorrhage into the tumor may cause sudden severe abdominal pain due to stretching of the tumor capsule. If primary tumors arise from the organ of Zuckerkandl, bladder and bowel symptoms may also be seen due to direct compression.

Primary thoracic tumors may be discovered as incidental findings or can be asymptomatic. Higher thoracic and cervical masses can also lead to Horner's syndrome (associated with unilateral ptosis, miosis and anhidrosis), superior vena cava syndrome or respiratory distress due to pressure on surrounding structures.

Paraspinal tumors can also have epidural or intradural extension and can cause symptoms from compression of nerve roots and spinal cord. These symptoms can include paraplegia, bladder or bowel dysfunction or radicular nerve pain. Spinal cord compression can become a medical emergency in some patients with neuroblastoma (**Table 1**).

http://dx.doi.org/10.5772/intechopen.70486

Location of tumor or area of metastatic involvement	Signs and symptoms
Abdomen/pelvis	Distension, constipation, urinary retention, pain, hypertension (due to renal vein compression)
Thorax	Respiratory distress, superior vena cava syndrome, Horner's syndrome
Neck	Swelling
Presacral/paraspinal tumors	Urinary retention, paraplegia/paresis, clonus
Metastases	Bone pain, irritability, cytopenias (anemia causing pallor, petechiae), periorbital ecchymoses, weight loss, fever
4S/4M metastases	Hepatomegaly, hyperbilirubinemia, coagulopathy, bluish skin nodules, respiratory distress due to abdominal distension
Paraneoplastic syndromes	VIP secreting tumors: intractable diarrhea OMS: myoclonic jerking and random eye movements

Table 1. Neuroblastoma symptomatology.

2.2. Metastatic disease

Approximately half of the patients present with metastasis. Metastasis can be lymphatic or hematogenous. Distant metastatic sites include cortex of bones, bone marrow, liver and non-contiguous lymph nodes. Neuroblastoma usually spreads to metaphyseal, skull and orbital bones. This can hence lead to symptoms of periorbital ecchymosis (raccoon eyes), proptosis and visual impairment. Children with metastatic tumors can be quite ill appearing at presentation as opposed to the relative benign nature of presentation of children with localized disease and can have fever, generalized body pain (due to bony metastases), weight loss and irritability. Other sites of distant metastasis can be in the lungs or intracranial. Clinical syndromes or paraneoplastic syndromes known to be associated with the presentation of neuroblastoma are summarized in **Table 2**.

2.3. Stage 4S neuroblastoma

The strikingly different phenotype of neuroblastoma is called 4S (S: special). It is a unique presentation of neuroblastoma seen in infants. This is seen to occur in about 5% cases of neuroblastoma [18]. These infants usually have small localized primary tumors; however have diffuse metastatic involvement at presentation. Metastatic sites can include diffuse involvement of liver, hepatomegaly, sometimes significant enough to cause respiratory compromise, diffuse subcutaneous nodules due to metastasis to skin, metastases to the bone marrow.

2.4. Paraneoplastic syndromes

There are two well described, but rare paraneoplastic syndromes associated with neuroblastoma, secretory diarrhea (due to production of vasoactive intestinal peptide from the tumor) and opsoclonus myoclonus ataxia syndrome (OMS). OMS consists of opsoclonus

Eponym	Features associated with syndrome
Pepper syndrome	Involvement of the liver with metastatic disease with or without respiratory distress
Horner syndrome	Unilateral ptosis, myosis, and anhydrosis associated with a thoracic or cervical primary tumor. Symptoms tend to persist following tumor resection
Hutchinson syndrome	Limping and irritability in young child seen with bone and bone marrow metastases
Opsoclonus mycoclonus ataxia syndrome	Random eye movement and myoclonic jerking in the presence or absence of cerebellar ataxia. Usually associated with a biologically favorable and differentiated tumor. The condition is thought to be immune mediated. It may not resolve with tumor removal, and exhibits progressive neuropsychological sequelae
Kerner-Morrison syndrome	Intractable secretory diarrhea due to tumor secretion of vasointestinal peptides
Neurocristopathy syndrome	Neuroblastoma associated with other neural crest disorders, including congenital hypoventilation syndrome or Hirshprung disease. Germline mutations in the paired homeobox gene PHOX2B have been identified in a subset of such patients

Adapted from Ref. [57]. For references, please refer to text.

Table 2. Syndromes associated with neuroblastoma.

(conjugate, multidirectional, chaotic eye movements), myoclonus (non-epileptic limb jerking) and ataxia (loss of balance). Between 1 and 3% of patients with neuroblastoma can have OMS [28, 29]. In most patients, the syndrome itself leads to the diagnosis of neuroblastoma; however it may rarely occur after tumor resection or even at relapse. In at least half of the children affected, OMS is associated with underlying occult or clinically apparent neur oblastoma. Hence, a thorough diagnostic evaluation for neuroblastoma at presentation is necessary in all patients with OMS, after exclusion of central nervous system pathology. A few previously reported series [28, 30, 31] show that 90% of patients presenting with OMS were without metastases at diagnosis, compared to 40–50% with metastases in non-OMS patients. OMS is thought to be due to an antineural antibody that cross-reacts with the antigen on both neuroblastoma and the normal nervous system tissue. Tumor biology, including MYCN copy number and Shimada histopathologic classification are usually favorable in OMS patients, which correlates with the excellent survival rate found in patients with OMS and neuroblastoma [28].

Treatment has been documented with various agents including glucocorticoids, adrenocorticotrophic hormone and intravenous immunoglobulin [29]. However almost 80% of patients will experience relapse of symptoms with weaning of treatment measures or with a viral syndrome. OMS can also be associated with long term chronic neurological complications.

Treatment resistant secretory diarrhea is seen in approximately 4% of patients with neuroblastoma and thought to be due to overproduction of vasoactive intestinal peptide (VIP) by maturing neuroblastoma cells [32, 33]. It is associated with chronic watery diarrhea and failure to thrive. It usually resolves after surgical removal of the primary tumor.

3. Diagnosis

3.1. Diagnostic criteria

Diagnosis of neuroblastoma is most commonly established from histopathologic evaluation of the primary tumor tissue. Most cases can be differentiated based on hematoxylin and eosin staining especially if features of neuronal differentiation are present. In case of minimal differentiation, immunohistochemical staining for neuron-specific enolase, chromogranin A and/or synaptophysin are used.

Diagnosis of neuroblastoma can also be established by a combination of tumor cells detected in the bone marrow and elevated catecholamines or their metabolites [vanillylmandelic acid (VMA), homovanillic acid (HVA) and dopamine]. Urinary VMA and HVA should both be measured for diagnostic purposes and for undifferentiated tumors dopamine may be measured.

3.2. Clinical disease assessment

Clinical evaluation of disease includes cross-sectional imaging of the primary tumor by magnetic resonance imaging (MRI) or computed tomography (CT). This imaging determines the size of the primary tumor, regional extent of the disease, distant metastatic spread to neck, chest, abdomen and pelvis. Bilateral bone marrow biopsies are required to assess for presence of tumor cells in the bone marrow. Radioiodine labeled metaiodobenzylguanidine (MIBG) is a nonrepinephrine analog that selectively concentrates in sympathetic nervous tissues. It can be used to detect primary tumor as well as detect occult soft tissue disease in addition to osteomedullary disease [34]. In the scenario that MIBG is unavailable, technetium bone scan can also be used to detect bony metastases (however is not as sensitive or specific as MIBG). Bone scan or FDG-PET scan are used to assess metastatic disease in patients whose tumors are not MIBG avid.

4. Staging and risk stratification

4.1. Staging

Until recently, the criteria for staging at diagnosis were based on the International Neuroblastoma Staging System (INSS) as shown in **Table 3** [35]. INSS stages 1–3 have localized tumors classified based on the amount of resection, invasion and nodal involvement. Stage 4 is defined as distant metastases; 4S is characterized by metastases to the liver, skin, and/or marrow in infants and is usually associated with favorable biological features and can undergo spontaneous regression.

In 2009, the International Neuroblastoma Risk Group's (INRG) stratification system was developed by a major consortium of North America, Europe, Japan, and Australia. The INRG

Stage	Description of disease and extension
1	Localized tumor with complete gross excision, with or without microscopic residual disease representative ipsilateral lymph nodes negative for tumor microscopically (nodes attached to and removed with the primary tumor may be positive)
2A	Localized tumor with incomplete gross resection; representative ipsilateral nonadherent lymph nodes negative for tumor microscopically
2B	Localized tumor with or without complete gross excision, with ipsilateral nonadherent lymph nodes positive for tumor; enlarged contralateral lymph nodes must be negative microscopically
3	Unresectable unilateral tumor infiltrating across the midline*, with or without regional lymph node involvement; or localized unilateral tumor with contralateral regional lymph node involvement; or midline tumor with bilateral extension by infiltration (unresectable) or by lymph node involvement
4	Any primary tumor with dissemination to distant lymph nodes, bone, bone marrow, liver, skin, and/or other organs (except as defined for stage 4S)
4S	Localized primary tumor (as defined for stage 1, 2A or 2B) with dissemination limited to skin, liver, and/or bone marrow# (limited to infants <1 year of age)

*The midline is the vertebral column. Tumors originating on one side and crossing the midline must infiltrate to or beyond the opposite side of the vertebral column.

#Marrow involvement in 4S should be minimal (<10% of total nucleated cells identified as malignant on bone marrow aspirate or biopsy). More extensive marrow involvement is stage 4.

Data adapted from Ref. [58].

Table 3. International Neuroblastoma Risk Group Staging System (INSS).

staging system is based on imaging criteria and the extent of locoregional disease is determined by the presence or absence of image-defined risk factors. And the extent of locoregional disease is determined by the presence or absence of image-defined risk factors [36] as shown in **Table 4**.

4.2. Risk stratification

Neuroblastoma is classified into low risk, intermediate risk, and high risk based on multiple factors including clinical and biological factors that have been shown to predict prognosis and the risk of recurrence. These factors include age, stage, histology, DNA index, and MYCN amplification (MYCNA) and are used to assign treatment groups by the Children's Oncology Group [1]. The INRG developed classification system defines similar cohorts using the INRG database of 8800 patients treated between 1990 and 2002. This now helps facilitate comparisons across international clinical trials (**Table 5**) [37].

4.2.1. Prognostic variables of neuroblastoma

Multiple variables are used for risk prediction and as prognostic markers of neuroblastoma. The most commonly used prognostic markers used in all cooperative groups are discussed here.

Stage: Stage of the disease using the INSS system has been correlated with patient outcome and used by all cooperative groups to risk stratify. Most patients with INSS stage 1 are cured by surgery alone, and most patients with stage 4 require highly intensive, multimodality therapy.

For the stages in between, therapy is based on other biologic factors. As the genetic and biologic characteristics of neuroblastoma are better defined, we will likely rely more on them and less on the disease stage or histology.

Ipsilateral tumor extension within two body compartments
Neck-chest, chest-abdomen, abdomen-pelvis
Neck
Encases carotid and/or vertebral artery and/or internal jugular vein; extends to skull base; compresses trachea
Cervicothoracic junction
Encases brachial plexus roots or subclavian vessels and/or vertebral or carotid artery; compresses trachea
Thorax
Encases the aorta and/or major branches; compresses trachea and/or principal bronchi; lower mediastinal tumor infiltrating costovertebral junction between T9 and 12
Thoracoabdominal
Encases the aorta and/or vena cava
Abdomen/pelvis
Infiltrates the porta hepatis and/or the hepatoduodenal ligament; encases branches of the superior mesenteric artery at the mesenteric root or origin of celiac axis and/or superior mesenteric artery; invades one or both renal pedicles; encases aorta and/or vena cava or iliac vessels, crossing sciatic notch
Intraspinal tumor extension whatever the location provided that
More than one-third of the spinal canal in the axial plane invaded and/or the perimedullary leptomeningeal spaces not visible and/or the spinal cord signal abnormal
Infiltration of adjacent organs/structures
Pericardium, diaphragm, kidney, liver, duodeno-pancreatic block, and mesentery IDRFs are used to determine the ability to completely resect locoregional tumors at diagnosis based on surgical risk factors that can be defined by IDRFs detected on cross-sectional imaging with CT and/or MRI

Data adapted from Ref. [59].

Table 4. Image defined risk factors.

Stage	Description
L1	Localized tumor not involving vital structures as defined by the list of image-defined risk factors and confined to one body compartment
L2	Locoregional tumor with presence of one or more IDRFs
M	Distant metastatic disease (except stage MS)
MS	Metastatic disease in children younger than 18 mo. with metastases confined to skin, liver, and/or bone marrow

Data adapted from Ref. [59].

Table 5. International risk group staging system (INRGSS).

INRG stage	Age (months)	Histology	Grade of tumor differentiation	*MYCN*	11q aberration	Ploidy	Pretreatment risk group
L1/L2		GN maturing, GNB intermixed					Very low
L1		Any, except GN maturing or GNB intermixed					Very low High
L2	<18 M	Any, except GN maturing or GNB intermixed		NA	No Yes		Low Intermediate
	>=18M	GNB nodular neuroblastoma	Differentiating	NA	No Yes		Low Intermediate
			Poorly differentiated or undifferentiated	NA Amplified			Intermediate high
M	<18			NA		HD	Low
	<12			NA		D	Intermediate
	12–<18			NA		D	Intermediate
	<18			Amplified			High
	>=18						High
MS	<18			NA	No Yes		Very low High
							High

Classification schema is based on analysis of 8800 patients in the INRG database (1990–2002). Risk groups are very low risk (5-year event-free survival [EFS] >85%); low risk (5-year EFS >75–85%); IR (5-year EFS 50–75%); HR (5-year EFS <50%).

Abbreviations: GN: ganglioneuroma; GNB: ganglioneuroblastoma; INRG: International Neuroblastoma Risk Group; NA: not amplified; HD: hyperdiploid; D: diploid.

Adapted from Ref. [60].

Table 6. International Neuroblastoma Risk Group pretreatment classification scheme.

Age: Age was one of the first and most important prognostic factors identified. Patients younger than 18 months of age have a much better prognosis compared to the older patients [38, 39], especially for patients between 12 and 18 months of age with biologically favorable disease. Older children, adolescents and young adults have a more indolent course and far worse outcomes [40].

Pathology: Shimada proposed a histology-based classification of tumors into "favorable" and "unfavorable" by combining age with extent of tumor differentiation, Schwannian components in tumor and degree of mitosis [1].

Biologic factors: Current risk stratification for neuroblastoma includes *MYCN* copies by fluorescent in situ hybridization, DNA ploidy by flow cytometry and tumor histology. *MYCNA* (*MYCN* amplification) is defined as greater than 10 copies and is detected in almost 20% of neuroblastoma tumors with a higher incidence in INSS stages 3 and 4, but only 5% of stages

1, 2 and 4S [36]. Multiple studies so far have demonstrated that patients with *MYCNA* have a significantly worse outcome [14, 15, 41].

A systematic review from a literature search of prognostic tumor markers in neuroblastoma was published, and reported 31 important prognostic factors each reported in five or more papers [42]. Meta-analysis of these markers showed that MYCN and DNA ploidy had the strongest prognostic impact. Most neuroblastomas have a nuclear DNA content in the diploid range. Tumors from patients who have lower stages of disease will often be hyperdiploid (DNA index > 1) or near triploid. DNA content is most significant as a prognostic marker in infants and patients with localized disease [1]. Other most commonly deleted chromosomal regions in neuroblastoma include 1p, 4p, 11q, 14q. Recurrent mutations are not frequent in neuroblastoma. Hence the identification of genes and signaling pathways with altered expression continue to be discovered and used to add additional value to prognostic factors and therapeutic targets involved in neuroblastoma apoptosis, drug resistance, angiogenesis, metastasis and inflammation [3, 43].

These factors were then combined to form a pre-treatment Risk Group Stratification as shown in **Table 6**.

5. Conventional treatment of neuroblastoma

The diagnosis and treatment of neuroblastoma is a multidisciplinary approach. Risk stratification is the first and most important step of treatment planning. It includes surgical biopsy especially to assess tumor genetic and histologic features, most importantly in patients less than 18 months with metastatic disease.

5.1. Treatment of low and intermediate risk neuroblastoma

Patients with low- or intermediate-risk neuroblastoma have excellent outcomes, and a series of cooperative group trials evaluating reductions in therapy using risk-based treatment approaches for these children has led to decreased therapy-related toxicities and improved outcomes. Survival rates for patients with INSS stage 1 disease are excellent with surgery alone and rare recurrences can be cured easily with salvage chemotherapy [44]. Survival rate for these groups with surgery alone is as high as 95%. For patients with INSS stage 1, 2A, 2B chemotherapy is reserved for patients with localized neuroblastoma with life threatening symptoms, or even for patients who experience recurrence or progressive disease.

Stage 4S neuroblastoma without MYCNA, undergo spontaneous regression. Chemotherapy or even low dose radiation can be used for large tumors causing symptoms or massive hepatomegaly [45].

Patients with intermediate risk disease which includes patients with INSS stage 3 and infants with stage 4/M and favorable biologic features are treated with regimens using surgical resection and moderate dose chemotherapy as the backbone. Patients with favorable tumor characteristics including infants with stage 4/M without MYCNA, the survival rates for surgery combined with moderate dose chemotherapy is greater than 90% [46].

5.2. Treatment of high risk neuroblastoma

Current treatment strategies for high risk neuroblastoma consist of three phases: induction phase, which consists of removal of gross tumor and achieving local control. The second phase of consolidation is to treat remaining chemotherapy-exposed cells to achieve lowest possible residual disease. Post-consolidation or maintenance phase is finally for treatment of the minimal residual disease. A general overview of the current day standard of care treatment strategy is described in **Figure 1**.

5.2.1. Induction therapy

Standard Children's Oncology Group (COG) induction regimens include various combinations of alkylators, anthracyclines, topoisomerase I and II inhibitors, platinum compounds delivered in 21 day cycles for 5–6 cycles. A successful induction which leads to complete remission (CR) or very good partial remission (VGPR) has been shown to correlate with improved overall survival. Following five cycles of induction chemotherapy, local control of primary tumor site is achieved with a combination of aggressive surgical resection and radiation therapy to the surgical bed. Surgery is performed after four to six cycles of induction chemotherapy to improve resectability and minimize surgery related complications. Complete tumor resection appears to correlate with improved local control and also significantly improved event-free survival (EFS) [47].

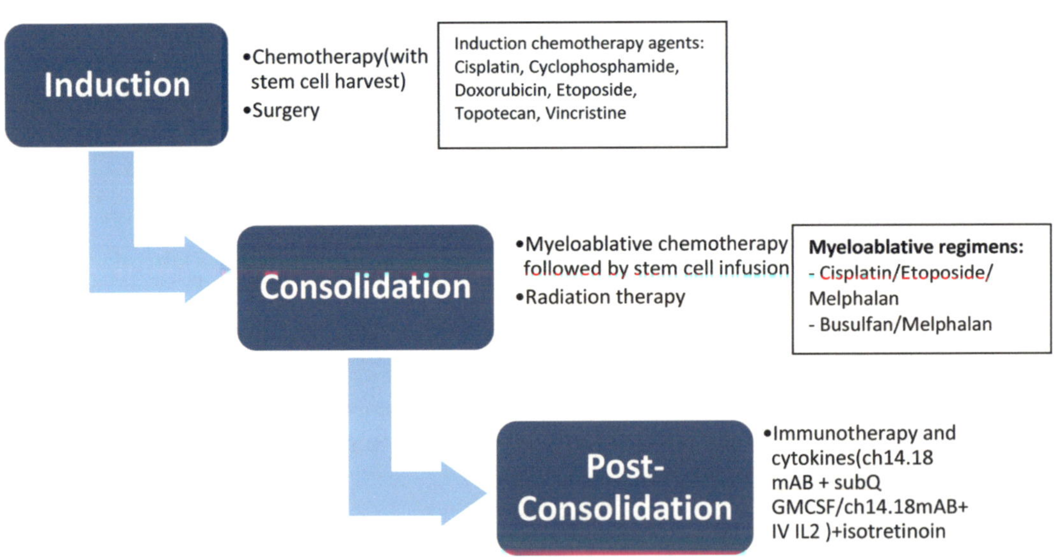

Figure 1. Treatment strategy currently used for patients with high risk neuroblastoma. ch14.18: chimeric 14.18, mAB: monoclonal antibody, GMCSF: granulocyte-macrophage colony stimulating factor, IL-2: interleukin-2.

5.2.2. Consolidation therapy

Several clinical trials performed in North America, Germany and Europe over the past 20 years has demonstrated improved outcomes following myeloablative therapy with autologous stem cell rescue. A Cochrane systems meta-analysis review by Yalçin et al. revealed that myeloablative chemotherapy has improved EFS [48]. The North American groups have traditionally used cyclophosphamide/etoposide/Melphalan for chemotherapy, whereas the European group (SIOPEN) data results suggest that patients randomized to the Busulfan/Melphalan arm had superior outcomes [49]. Another Children's Oncology Group Study ANBL0532 also studied differences in outcomes between patients receiving single vs tandem myeloablative transplants (**Figure 2**) and found that 3-year event-free survival was significantly better in the tandem group than in the single group (61.4% vs 48.4%; $P = 0.0081$). There was a nonsignificant trend toward better 3-year overall survival in the tandem group than in the single group before immunotherapy (74.0% vs 69.1%; $P = 0.1850$).

Consolidation therapy also consists of radiation to the primary site, as neuroblastoma is one of the most radio-sensitive pediatric tumors. Doses of 2160 cGy (centiGray) in daily 180 cGy fractions to the primary sites decreases local recurrence rates [50]. Radiation is also delivered to MIBG-avid metastatic sites, with a recent report suggesting that non-irradiated lesions have a higher risk of involvement at the time of relapse [51].

5.2.3. Post-consolidation biologic and immunotherapies

Following surgery and high dose chemotherapy followed by autologous stem cell rescue, treatment with synthetic retinoid isotretinoin (cis-retinoic acid) showed significantly promising

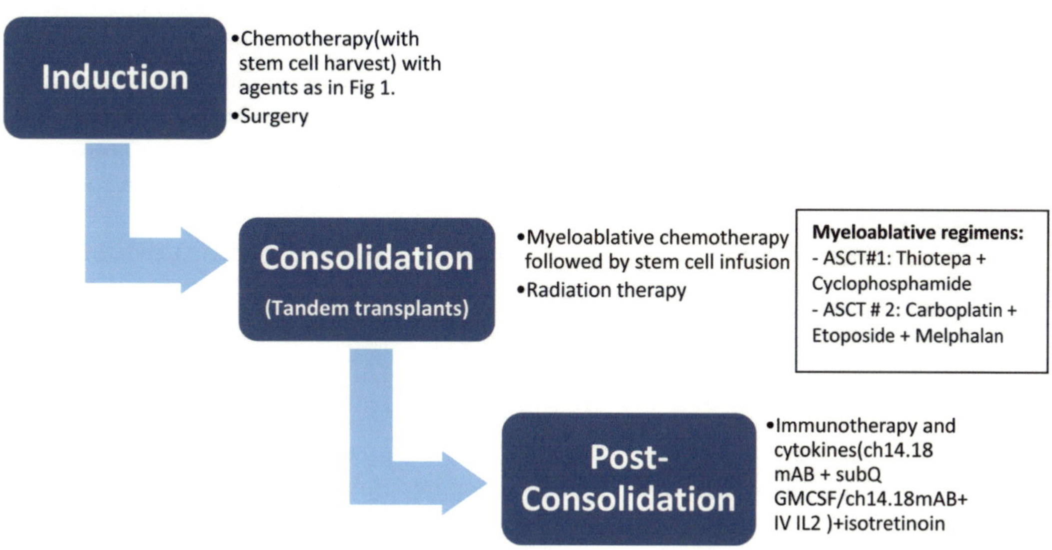

Figure 2. Tandem autologous stem cell transplant regimen used for patients with high risk neuroblastoma. ASCT: autologous stem cell transplant, ch14.18: chimeric 14.18, mAB: monoclonal antibody, GMCSF: granulocyte-macrophage colony stimulating factor, IL-2: interleukin-2.

results and is hence an established as standard of care [52]. Another randomized control trial also demonstrated that the addition of anti-GD2 chimeric monoclonal antibody (mAB) with cytokines (granulocyte-macrophage colony stimulating factor and interleukin 2) improved survival [53]. Additional studies have also shown the benefit of immunotherapy at diagnosis as well as first recurrence of disease. However this regimen has multiple side effects: fever, allergic reactions, hypotension, pain, capillary leak syndrome.

In spite of all the therapeutic modalities explained above directed at high risk neuroblastoma, even-free survival for these patients is only 40–50%. In the INRG data set, overall survival for patients who relapse after treatment for low/intermediate risk disease was 65%, 5 years after recurrence, but for patients with high risk/metastatic disease, the 5-year overall survival was only 8% after recurrence. There is hence a real need for potential new targeted therapy and also alternative therapies to improve chemo-sensitivity in these patients with high risk neuroblastoma.

6. Novel therapeutic interventions

Relapse strategies are divided into chemotherapy, immunotherapy, MIBG/radioisotopes and targeted therapies. These therapies are mostly being tested in Phase I and II trials in patients with recurrent or relapsed neuroblastoma.

6.1. Immunotherapeutic targets

Due to the initial success of passive immunotherapy with anti-GD2 antibody chimeric 14.18 in high risk neuroblastoma, there has been a surge in the development of additional immunotherapeutic modalities. Clinical trials evaluating anti-GD2 therapeutics and chemotherapy (irinotecan plus temozolomide; COG ANBL1221) or the immunostimulatory molecule lenalidomide are under way. Additional pilot studies evaluating monoclonal antibody 1A7 as a surrogate GD2 vaccine and active immunization against GD2 and GD3 combined with the immunostimulant beta-glucan in patients with complete or very good partial remission have shown encouraging results. There is also increasing interest in chimeric antigen receptor expressing autologous T cells for cellular-based therapy in neuroblastoma [54]. In addition to chimeric T cells, infusions of natural killer cells, dendritic cells are also under investigation, especially in patients with relapsed disease.

6.2. Targeted radiotherapy

^{131}I-mIBG (^{131}Iodized- metaiodobenzylguanidine) is a beta particle-emitting norepinephrine analog which is taken up by cells expressing the norepinephrine transporter. It has been one of the earliest and most successful therapies for relapsed neuroblastoma. ^{131}I-mIBG has the properties of excellent tumor targeting, the potential of delivering high levels of absorbed radiation to tumors in soft tissue, bone and bone marrow. It is also rapidly cleared by the kidneys, hence making it an ideal therapeutic agent in mIBG-avid neuroblastoma and pheochromocytoma. Previously, studied as an agent in patients with relapsed or refractory disease, it is now being incorporated as part of induction therapy in those with mIBG-avid neuroblastoma. After years of being studied to establish safety and efficacy, ^{131}I-mIBG therapies is now being studied in combination with other chemotherapy agents, radio sensitizers, hyperbaric oxygen, gene therapy or ionizing radiation from external beam radiation. A brilliant review of this subject is presented in the article by Streby et al. [55]. A recent Children's Oncology Group Study is investigating the effects of administering ^{131} I-mIBG in combination with induction chemotherapy (in patients with mIBG sensitive tumors at diagnosis).

6.3. Molecular guided targeted therapy

Several potential molecular targets and inhibitors are now being tested especially in preclinical and Phase I trials. A small subset of ALK aberrant tumors can be targeted with ALK inhibitors [16]. For patients harboring *MYCNA*, preclinical studies are suggestive of bromodomain and extraterminal domain inhibitors (BET inhibitors) inducing cell death by interfering with *MYCN* transcription [56].

Other agents that target cell cycle, angiogenesis and cell differentiation are also currently under investigation and awaiting further preclinical and preliminary clinical studies.

Due to the variety of therapy options that are under study, it appears that most future clinical trials will incorporate a salient novel agent in combination with common chemotherapy as backbone regimens.

Author details

Neema Bhat* and Lisa McGregor

*Address all correspondence to: neema.bhat@outlook.com

Penn State Health Center, Hershey, Pennsylvania, USA

References

[1] Irwin MS, Park JR. Neuroblastoma: Paradigm for precision medicine. Pediatric Clinics of North America. 2015 Feb;**62**(1):225-256

[2] Park JR, Bagatell R, London WB, Maris JM, Cohn SL, Mattay KK, et al. Children's Oncology Group's 2013 blueprint for research: Neuroblastoma. Pediatric Blood & Cancer. 2013 Jun;**60**(6):985-993

[3] Cheung N-KV, Dyer MA. Neuroblastoma: Developmental biology, cancer genomics and immunotherapy. Nature Reviews Cancer. 2013 Jun;**13**(6):397-411

[4] Dhir S, Wheeler K. Neonatal neuroblastoma. Early Human Development. 2010 Oct;**86**(10): 601-605

[5] Heck JE, Ritz B, Hung RJ, Hashibe M, Boffetta P. The epidemiology of neuroblastoma: A review. Paediatric and Perinatal Epidemiology. 2009 Mar;**23**(2):125-143

[6] Johnson KA, Aplenc R, Bagatell R. Survival by race among children with extracranial solid tumors in the United States between 1985 and 2005. Pediatric Blood & Cancer. 2011 Mar;**56**(3):425-431

[7] Speleman F, Park JR, Henderson TO. Neuroblastoma: A tough nut to crack. American Society of Clinical Oncology educational book. American Society of Clinical Oncology. Meeting. 2016;**35**:e548-e557

[8] Mossé YP, Laudenslager M, Longo L, Cole KA, Wood A, Attiyeh EF, et al. Identification of ALK as a major familial neuroblastoma predisposition gene. Nature. 2008 Oct 16;**455**(7215):930-935

[9] Molenaar JJ, Domingo-Fernández R, Ebus ME, Lindner S, Koster J, Drabek K, et al. LIN28B induces neuroblastoma and enhances MYCN levels via let-7 suppression. Nature Genetics. 2012 Nov;**44**(11):1199-1206

[10] Schwab M, Alitalo K, Klempnauer KH, Varmus HE, Bishop JM, Gilbert F, et al. Amplified DNA with limited homology to myc cellular oncogene is shared by human neuroblastoma cell lines and a neuroblastoma tumour. Nature. 1983 Sep 15;**305**(5931):245-248

[11] Schwab M, Varmus HE, Bishop JM, Grzeschik KH, Naylor SL, Sakaguchi AY, et al. Chromosome localization in normal human cells and neuroblastomas of a gene related to c-myc. Nature. 1984 Mar 15;**308**(5956):288-291

[12] Seeger RC, Brodeur GM, Sather H, Dalton A, Siegel SE, Wong KY, et al. Association of multiple copies of the N-myc oncogene with rapid progression of neuroblastomas. The New England Journal of Medicine. 1985 Oct 31;**313**(18):1111-1116

[13] Schmidt ML, Lukens JN, Seeger RC, Brodeur GM, Shimada H, Gerbing RB, et al. Biologic factors determine prognosis in infants with stage IV neuroblastoma: A prospective Children's Cancer Group study. Journal of Clinical Oncology : Official Journal of the American Society of Clinical Oncology. 2000 Mar;**18**(6):1260-1268

[14] Maris JM, Hogarty MD, Bagatell R, Cohn SL. Neuroblastoma. The Lancet London England. 2007 Jun 23;**369**(9579):2106-2120

[15] Huang M, Weiss WA. Neuroblastoma and MYCN. Cold Spring Harbor Perspectives in Medicine. 2013 Oct 1;**3**(10):a014415

[16] Carpenter EL, Mossé YP. Targeting ALK in neuroblastoma–Preclinical and clinical advancements. Nature Reviews. Clinical Oncology. 2012 May 15;**9**(7):391-399

[17] Mossé YP, Lim MS, Voss SD, Wilner K, Ruffner K, Laliberte J, et al. Safety and activity of crizotinib for paediatric patients with refractory solid tumours or anaplastic large-cell lymphoma: A Children's Oncology Group phase 1 consortium study. The Lancet Oncology. 2013 May;**14**(6):472-480

[18] Pizzo PA PD. Neuroblastoma. In: Principles and Practice of Pediatric Oncology. 7th ed. Philadelphia: Lippincott Williams & Wilkins; 2016. pp. 777-778

[19] Kushner BH, Gilbert F, Helson L. Familial neuroblastoma. Case reports, literature review, and etiologic considerations. Cancer. 1986 May 1;**57**(9):1887-1893

[20] Rohrer T, Trachsel D, Engelcke G, Hammer J. Congenital central hypoventilation syndrome associated with Hirschsprung's disease and neuroblastoma: Case of multiple neurocristopathies. Pediatric Pulmonology. 2002 Jan;**33**(1):71-76

[21] Bissig H, Staehelin F, Tolnay M, Avoledo P, Richter J, Betts D, et al. Co-occurrence of neuroblastoma and nephroblastoma in an infant with Fanconi's anemia. Human Pathology. 2002 Oct;**33**(10):1047-1051

[22] Perri P, Longo L, McConville C, Cusano R, Rees SA, Seri M, et al. Linkage analysis in families with recurrent neuroblastoma. Annals of the New York Academy of Sciences. 2002 Jun;**963**:74-84

[23] Perri P, Bachetti T, Longo L, Matera I, Seri M, Tonini GP, et al. PHOX2B mutations and genetic predisposition to neuroblastoma. Oncogene. 2005 Apr 21;**24**(18):3050-3053

[24] Janoueix-Lerosey I, Lequin D, Brugières L, Ribeiro A, de Pontual L, Combaret V, et al. Somatic and germline activating mutations of the ALK kinase receptor in neuroblastoma. Nature. 2008 Oct 16;**455**(7215):967-970

[25] Rossbach H-C, Baschinsky D, Wynn T, Obzut D, Sutcliffe M, Tebbi C. Composite adrenal anaplastic neuroblastoma and virilizing adrenocortical tumor with germline TP53 R248W mutation. Pediatric Blood & Cancer. 2008 Mar;**50**(3):681-683

[26] Birch JM, Alston RD, McNally RJ, Evans DG, Kelsey AM, Harris M, et al. Relative frequency and morphology of cancers in carriers of germline TP53 mutations. Oncogene. 2001 Aug 2;**20**(34):4621-4628

[27] Reid S, Schindler D, Hanenberg H, Barker K, Hanks S, Kalb R, et al. Biallelic mutations in PALB2 cause Fanconi anemia subtype FA-N and predispose to childhood cancer. Nature Genetics. 2007 Feb;**39**(2):162-164

[28] Matthay KK, Blaes F, Hero B, Plantaz D, De Alarcon P, Mitchell WG, et al. Opsoclonus myoclonus syndrome in neuroblastoma a report from a workshop on the dancing eyes syndrome at the advances in neuroblastoma meeting in Genoa, Italy, 2004. Cancer Letters. 2005 Oct 18;**228**(1-2):275-282

[29] Gorman MP. Update on diagnosis, treatment, and prognosis in opsoclonus-myoclonus-ataxia syndrome. Current Opinion in Pediatrics. 2010 Dec;**22**(6):745-750

[30] Krug P, Schleiermacher G, Michon J, Valteau-Couanet D, Brisse H, Peuchmaur M, et al. Opsoclonus-myoclonus in children associated or not with neuroblastoma. European Journal of Paediatric Neurology: EJPN: Official Journal of the European Paediatric Neurology Society. 2010 Sep;**14**(5):400-409

[31] Plantaz D, Michon J, Valteau-Couanet D, Coze C, Chastagner P, Bergeron C, et al. Opsoclonus-myoclonus syndrome associated with non-metastatic neuroblastoma. Long-term survival. Study of the French Society of Pediatric Oncologists. Archives de Pédiatrie Organe Officiel De La SociéTe FrançAise De PéDiatrie. 2000 Jun;**7**(6):621-628

[32] El Shafie M, Samuel D, Klippel CH, Robinson MG, Cullen BJ. Intractable diarrhea in children with VIP-secreting ganglioneuroblastomas. Journal of Pediatric Surgery. 1983 Feb;**18**(1):34-36

[33] Scheibel E, Rechnitzer C, Fahrenkrug J, Hertz H. Vasoactive intestinal polypeptide (VIP) in children with neural crest tumours. Acta Paediatrica Scandinavica. 1982 Sep;**71**(5):721-725

[34] Sharp SE, Trout AT, Weiss BD, Gelfand MJ. MIBG in neuroblastoma diagnostic imaging and therapy. Radiographics: A Review Publication of the Radiological Society of North America, Inc. 2016 Feb;**36**(1):258-278

[35] Park JR, Eggert A, Caron H. Neuroblastoma: Biology, prognosis, and treatment. Hematology/Oncology Clinics of North America. 2010 Feb;**24**(1):65-86

[36] Cohn SL, Pearson ADJ, London WB, Monclair T, Ambros PF, Brodeur GM, et al. The International Neuroblastoma Risk Group (INRG) classification system: An INRG Task Force report. Journal of Clinical Oncology: Official Journal of the American Society of Clinical Oncology. 2009 Jan 10;**27**(2):289-297

[37] Pinto NR, Applebaum MA, Volchenboum SL, Matthay KK, London WB, Ambros PF, et al. Advances in risk classification and treatment strategies for neuroblastoma. Journal of Clinical Oncology: Official Journal of the American Society of Clinical Oncology. 2015 Sep 20;**33**(27):3008-3017

[38] Schmidt ML, Lal A, Seeger RC, Maris JM, Shimada H, O'Leary M, et al. Favorable prognosis for patients 12 to 18 months of age with stage 4 nonamplified MYCN neuroblastoma: A Children's Cancer Group Study. Journal of Clinical Oncology: Official Journal of the American Society of Clinical Oncology. 2005 Sep 20;**23**(27):6474-6480

[39] George RE, London WB, Cohn SL, Maris JM, Kretschmar C, Diller L, et al. Hyperdiploidy plus nonamplified MYCN confers a favorable prognosis in children 12 to 18 months old with disseminated neuroblastoma: A Pediatric Oncology Group study. Journal of Clinical Oncology: Official Journal of the American Society of Clinical Oncology. 2005 Sep 20;**23**(27):6466-6473

[40] Mossé YP, Deyell RJ, Berthold F, Nagakawara A, Ambros PF, Monclair T, et al. Neuroblastoma in older children, adolescents and young adults: A report from the International Neuroblastoma Risk Group project. Pediatric Blood & Cancer. 2014 Apr;**61**(4):627-635

[41] Maris JM. Recent advances in neuroblastoma. The New England Journal of Medicine. 2010 Jun 10;**362**(23):2202-2211

[42] Vo KT, Matthay KK, Neuhaus J, London WB, Hero B, Ambros PF, et al. Clinical, biologic, and prognostic differences on the basis of primary tumor site in neuroblastoma: A report from the International Neuroblastoma Risk Group project. Journal of Clinical Oncology. 2014 Oct 1;**32**(28):3169-3176

[43] Cole KA, Maris JM. New strategies in refractory and recurrent neuroblastoma: Translational opportunities to impact patient outcome. Clinical Cancer Research: An Official Journal of the American Association for Cancer Research. 2012 May 1;**18**(9): 2423-2428

[44] Perez CA, Matthay KK, Atkinson JB, Seeger RC, Shimada H, Haase GM, et al. Biologic variables in the outcome of stages I and II neuroblastoma treated with surgery as primary therapy: A children's cancer group study. Journal of Clinical Oncology: Official Journal of the American Society of Clinical Oncology. 2000 Jan;**18**(1):18-26

[45] Nickerson HJ, Matthay KK, Seeger RC, Brodeur GM, Shimada H, Perez C, et al. Favorable biology and outcome of stage IV-S neuroblastoma with supportive care or minimal therapy: A Children's Cancer Group study. Journal of Clinical Oncology: Official Journal of the American Society of Clinical Oncology. 2000 Feb;**18**(3):477-486

[46] Meany HJ, London WB, Ambros PF, Matthay KK, Monclair T, Simon T, et al. Significance of clinical and biologic features in Stage 3 neuroblastoma: A report from the International Neuroblastoma Risk Group project. Pediatric Blood & Cancer. 2014 Nov;**61**(11):1932-1939

[47] von Allmen D, Davidoff AM, London WB, Van Ryn C, Haas-Kogan DA, Kreissman SG, et al. Impact of extent of resection on local control and survival in patients from the COG A3973 study with high-risk neuroblastoma. Journal of Clinical Oncology: Official Journal of the American Society of Clinical Oncology. 2017 Jan 10;**35**(2):208-216

[48] Yalçin B, Kremer LCM, van Dalen EC. High-dose chemotherapy and autologous haematopoietic stem cell rescue for children with high-risk neuroblastoma. Cochrane Database of Systematic Reviews. 2015 Oct **5**;(10):CD006301

[49] PL012 influence of surgical excision on survival of patients with high risk neuroblastoma. Report from Study 1 of Siop Europe (Siopen) Keith holmes, SIOPEN, London, United Kingdom

[50] Haas-Kogan DA, Swift PS, Selch M, Haase GM, Seeger RC, Gerbing RB, et al. Impact of radiotherapy for high-risk neuroblastoma: A Children's Cancer Group study. International Journal of Radiation Oncology, Biology, Physics. 2003 May 1;**56**(1):28-39

[51] Polishchuk AL, Li R, Hill-Kayser C, Little A, Hawkins RA, Hamilton J, et al. Likelihood of bone recurrence in prior sites of metastasis in patients with high-risk neuroblastoma. International Journal of Radiation Oncology, Biology, Physics. 2014 Jul 15;**89**(4):839-845

[52] Matthay KK, Reynolds CP, Seeger RC, Shimada H, Adkins ES, Haas-Kogan D, et al. Long-term results for children with high-risk neuroblastoma treated on a randomized trial of myeloablative therapy followed by 13-cis-retinoic acid: A children's oncology

group study. Journal of Clinical Oncology: Official Journal of the American Society of Clinical Oncology. 2009 Mar 1;**27**(7):1007-1013

[53] Yu AL, Gilman AL, Ozkaynak MF, London WB, Kreissman SG, Chen HX, et al. Anti-GD2 antibody with GM-CSF, interleukin-2, and isotretinoin for neuroblastoma. The New England Journal of Medicine. 2010 Sep 30;**363**(14):1324-1334

[54] Louis CU, Savoldo B, Dotti G, Pule M, Yvon E, Myers GD, et al. Antitumor activity and long-term fate of chimeric antigen receptor-positive T cells in patients with neuroblastoma. Blood. 2011 Dec 1;**118**(23):6050-6056

[55] Streby KA, Shah N, Ranalli MA, Kunkler A, Cripe TP. Nothing but NET: A review of norepinephrine transporter expression and efficacy of ^{131}I-mIBG therapy. Pediatric Blood & Cancer. 2015 Jan;**62**(1):5-11

[56] Henssen A, Althoff K, Odersky A, Beckers A, Koche R, Speleman F, et al. Targeting MYCN-driven transcription by BET-bromodomain inhibition. Clinical Cancer Research: An Official Journal of the American Association for Cancer Research. 2016 May 15;**22**(10):2470-2481

[57] Castleberry RP. Biology and treatment of neuroblastoma. Pediatric Clinics of North America. 1997;**44**:919-937

[58] Brodeur GM, Pritchard J, Berthold F, et al. Revisions of the international criteria for neuroblastoma diagnosis, staging, and response to treatment. Journal of Clinical Oncology. 1993;**11**(8):1466-1477

[59] Monclair T, Brodeur GM, Ambros PF, et al. The International Neuroblastoma Risk Group (INRG) staging system: An INRG task force report. Journal of Clinical Oncology. 2009;**27**(2):298-303

[60] Cohn SL, Pearson AD, London WB, et al. The International Neuroblastoma Risk Group [INRG] classification system: An INRG task force report. Journal of Clinical Oncology. 2009;**27**(2):295

Chapter 2

The Origin of Neuroblastoma

Gian Paolo Tonini

Additional information is available at the end of the chapter

http://dx.doi.org/10.5772/intechopen.69422

Abstract

It is widely accepted that neuroblastoma origin from Neural Crest Cells (NCC). NCC is a group of embryonic cells located in proximity to neural tube. During the embryonic development they migrate to generate the ganglia of sympathetic nervous system and the adrenal medulla. More than 50% of neuroblastoma masses are detected in the abdomen but the phases of tumorigenesis during the embryonic life are still unknown. Neuroblastoma cells show numerous copy number aberrations (CNAs), both numerical and structural. Several non-random CNAs are detected in clinical stage 4 and associated with tumor aggressiveness. On the contrary, neuroblastoma cells of infants or young patients have several numerical CNAs that are associated with a favorable outcome. *MYCN* oncogene amplification was one of the first genetic abnormalities observed in neuroblastoma and was found correlated to tumor aggressiveness. About 1% of all neuroblastoma show a hereditable fashion. Nowadays, the ALK gene has been discovered as predisposition gene for neuroblastoma. Moreover, thank to the genome-wide association studies, *BARD1*, *LMO1* and *LIN28* genes have been found linked to neuroblastoma predisposition. The two-step and multistep models are not satisfied the genesis of this tumor making the study of neuroblastoma tumorigenesis mandatory. Recently, the role of chromosome instability (CIN) became prominent to explain the neuroblastoma development. Indeed, the chromothripsis was observed in neuroblastoma cells of clinical stage 4, supporting the high genomic instability of these cells. The role of CIN in neuroblastoma is still unclear, but several experimental data suggest that CIN has a pivotal part in the genesis of neuroblastoma.

Keywords: neuroblastoma, neural crest cells, tumorigenesis, chromosomal instability, two-hit model, multistep model, chromosome instability

1. Introduction

The OMICs (the OMICs is a neologism referred to the study of: genomics, proteomics, transcriptomics, etc.) study of neuroblastoma has produced a huge amount of data generated by

INTECH
open science | open minds

© 2017 The Author(s). Licensee InTech. This chapter is distributed under the terms of the Creative Commons Attribution License (http://creativecommons.org/licenses/by/3.0), which permits unrestricted use, distribution, and reproduction in any medium, provided the original work is properly cited.

genomics profiling, gene expression and epigenetics analysis [1]. Nevertheless, these studies supply information about the picture of primary tumors or metastatic cells only at onset of the disease. More recently, Schramm et al. [2] were able to study the genome of neuroblastoma comparing the mutational profiling of tumor cells at onset of disease and at time of patient's relapse. This allowed the authors to investigate the tumor clonal evolution and demonstrate that new mutations were acquired during the tumor progression. Recurrent mutations in tumor of relapsed patients included: cadherin 5 (*CDH5*), dedicator of cytokinesis 8 (*DOCK8*), protein-tyrosine phosphatase nonreceptor type 4 (*PTPN14*), Harvey rat sarcoma viral oncogene homolog (*HRAS*) and Kirsten rat sarcoma viral oncogene homolog (*KRAS*), providing a lot of information concerning new mutations present in the tumor of patient at relapse. Since patient's relapse is a critical step in the cure of neuroblastoma for the reason that, usually, tumor is not responding to the therapy, it is reasonable that new mutations contribute to increase tumor aggressiveness and drug resistance. *MYCN* oncogene amplification is one of the most important gene abnormalities found in neuroblastoma, and it is largely used as tumor unfavorable marker. The *MYCN* status (normal versus amplified) is used to classify the relapse patient's risk. Consequently, in the last decade, in order to perform precision medicine, particular attention was focused to find mutations candidate to drug targeting [3].

However, although the OMICs approach allowed us to identify some new drugs useful for target therapy, the cure of neuroblastoma is partially ineffective with a 5-year overall survival of 35% [4].

Actually, the overall OMICs studies are lacking important information about the origin of neuroblastoma. Really, we do not know how and when the mutations that we observed are occurring in neuroblastoma cells. Some animal models have been produced to recapitulate the growth and development of neuroblastoma, and some mathematical models have been generated to mimic the tumorigenesis of the tumor, but the overall information about the genesis of neuroblastoma is still missing. Certainly, the deep knowledge about the neuroblastoma tumorigenesis will greatly contribute to the cure of this pediatric cancer.

2. From neural crest cell to neuroblastoma cell

There are evidences that neuroblastoma tumor cells originate from neural crest cell (NCC) [5, 6]. Most of neuroblastoma cells produce homovanillic acid and vanillylmandelic acid, two metabolites involved in catecholamine synthesis of sympathetic nervous system [7, 8].

The neuroblastoma is comprised in Neuroblastic Tumors a group of tumors with great heterogeneous morphology [9]. Neuroblastoma cells show small cell body with few cytoplasm and abundant nucleus, while some neuritis protrudes by the cell body. Neuroblastic Tumors are classified as: Neuroblastoma Schwannian stroma-poor (undifferentiated, poorly differentiated, differentiating), Ganglioneuroblastoma intermixed Schwannian stroma-rich and Ganglioneuroma. Undifferentiated Neuroblastoma Schwannian stroma-poor is one of the most aggressive Neuroblastic Tumors, whereas Ganglioneuroblastoma intermixed Schwannian stroma-rich and Ganglioneuroma are less aggressive. Ganglioneuroblastoma and Ganglioneuroma display heterogeneous morphology with large cells resembling ganglionic-like cells or Schwann-like cells. The latter are also identified as stromal cells. In **Figure 1**, the cell morphology of some Neuroblastic Tumors is shown.

It is also interesting to report that neuroblastoma cells of human-established cell lines produce a lot of long neuritis, creating a dense neural network after all-trans retinoid acid (ATRA) treatment [10, 11]. Moreover, the treatment with ATRA blocks the cellular proliferation inducing neuroblastoma cellular maturation. More than 50% of the patients onset with an abdominal mass, while other patients have head, neck and paraspinal infiltrated lymph-nodes [7]. Trunk NCC moves from dorsal to ventral region to form sympathetic ganglia and adrenal medulla.

It is still unclear if these cells are also a committee to become malignant neuroblastoma cells or if the malignant transformation is initiated after the NCC reached their final destination.

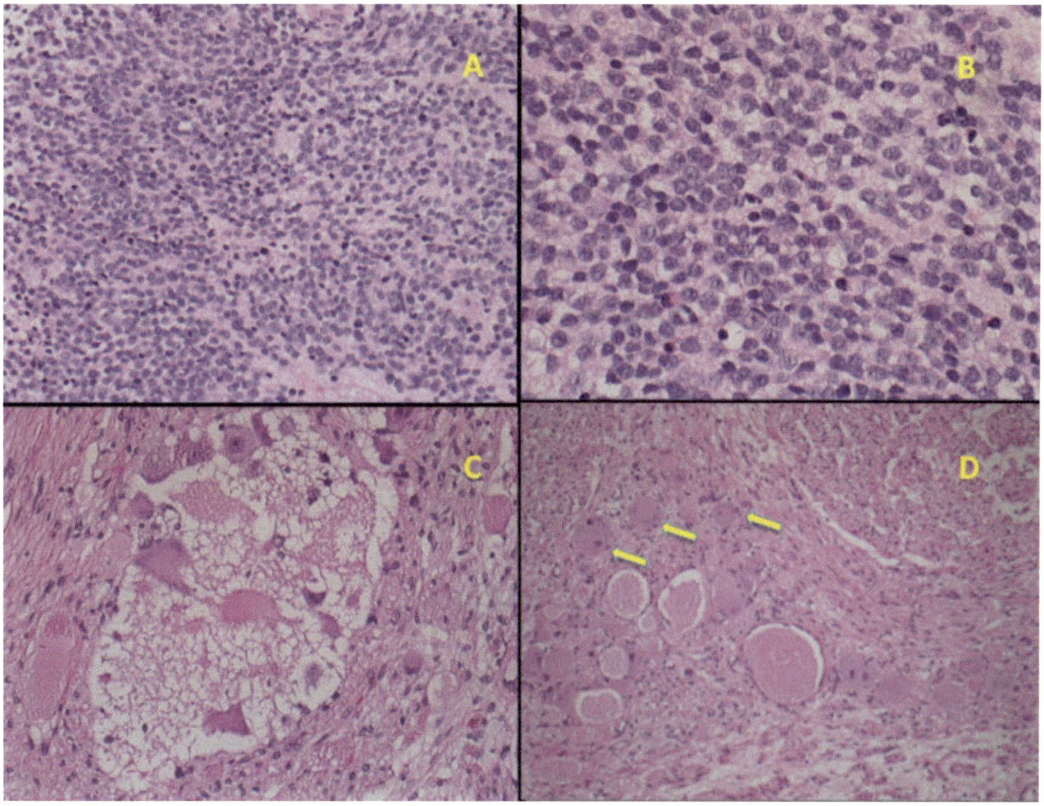

Figure 1. Morphological heterogeneity of neuroblastic tumors. (A) Poorly differentiated neuroblastoma stroma-poor (magnification 20x) and (B) same tumor (magnification 40x). Tumor tissue shows small blue cells with few cytoplasm and few stroma. (C) Ganglioneuroblastoma intermixed Schwannian stroma-rich (magnification 20x). Cells are embedded in abundant stroma. (D) Ganglioneuroma, very benign tumor; most of the tissue is stroma, and some ganglionic-like cells are visible (yellow arrow) (kindly provided by Dr. Luisa Santoro, University of Padua, Italy).

There are several evidences that neuroblastoma arises during fetal life. Ikeda et al. [12] have observed neuroblastoma cells in autoptic samples of infants. This observation clearly indicates that tumor may grow and develops during the fetal life. Patients with neuroblastoma stage 4S, a special group of patients that develop the tumor within one year of age and that may show onset of disease in the first month of life (**Figure 2**), are presumably developing the tumor already before birth. This has been demonstrated by Gigliotti et al. [13] who reported that six cases out of 45 stage 4S neuroblastomas were detected in utero. So that, we have several, indicating that neuroblastoma tumorigenesis may initiate during the fetal life.

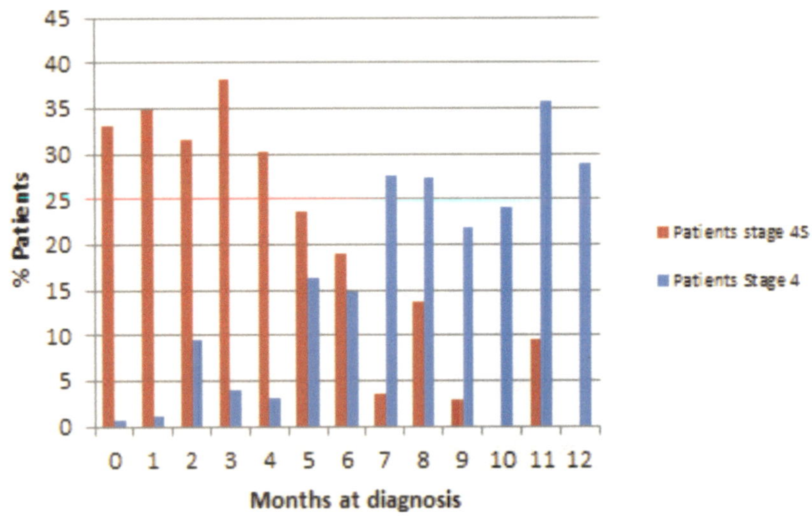

Figure 2. Distribution of stage 4S and stage 4 patients at onset during the first year of life. Most of stage 4S patients (red column) onset between 0 and 8 months, whereas patients at stage 4 (blue column) onset more frequently after 5 months [14].

3. Familial neuroblastoma and predisposition to neuroblastoma

About 1% of all neuroblastoma show familial cases. Genetic screenings of several families with recurrent neuroblastoma have shown that tumor is transmitted as recessive trait at low penetrance. In 2007, Longo et al. [14] have demonstrated a significant likelihood ratio for locus 2p by linkage analysis. Further, Mosse et al. [15] identified a locus at the chromosome region 2p23-24 with 104 genes that also included the *MYCN* gene. Next analysis showed significant mutations of Anaplastic Lymphoma Kinase (*ALK*) gene associated with the neuroblastoma predisposition. In neuroblastoma, *ALK* gene synthetizes the tyrosine alk receptor. Receptor autophosphorylation is promoted by mutation in kinase domain, and it is activating the alk pathway. Both germline and somatic *ALK* mutations were observed in neuroblastoma. Up to now, several mutations have been found in the kinase domain, but the most frequents are R1275 (43%), F1174 (30%) and F1245 (12%).

It is interesting to note that in human, both *MYCN* [16] and *ALK* [17] genes are highly expressed during the embryonic life and their expression decreases after the born. *MYCN* and *ALK* expression is not appreciable in the tissues of adult.

Recently, genome-wide association studies (GWAS) have been used to identify susceptibility gene variants in neuroblastoma. The GWAS studies are very useful to associate gene polymorphisms to tumor predisposition. Bosse et al. [18] identified the *BARD1 β*, an isoform of *BARD1* gene, associated with high-risk neuroblastoma. Oldridge et al. [19] found a polymorphism at locus of *LMO1* gene significantly associated with neuroblastoma susceptibility. In particular, they found the SNP rs 2168101, the variant most highly associated with the disease. A further association was found for *LIN28B* variants, making the *LIN28B* gene significantly involved in the neuroblastoma susceptibility [20].

4. Genomics and transcriptomics abnormalities in neuroblastoma cell

DNA content in neuroblastoma cells shows great variability. Most of the tumors with favorable evolution show triploid or near-triploid cells, whereas tumor of patients with unfavorable outcome shows diploid, near-diploid or tetraploid cells. Tumor of favorable cases has whole additional chromosomes and few structural damages, whereas tumor of patients with poor outcome usually has several nonrandom structural changes and few numerical chromosome aberrations [21–23].

Studies of neuroblastoma cell genome, by microarray comparative genomic hybridization, have shown the following nonrandom structural copy number aberrations (CNAs): deletions of chromosomes 1p36 region, 3p, 4p, 9p 11q 14q together gain of 1q, 2p24, 12p, 17q [21, 22, 24]. Structural CNAs are more frequently observed in tumor of patients with aggressive metastatic disease, and indeed, structural chromosome abnormalities are significantly associated with high tumor aggressiveness and disease progression [25]. This picture indicates that neuroblastoma cells have high chromosomal instability. Gain of chromosome 2p region is mainly due to the amplification of *MYCN* gene. The amplification of *MYCN* gene was discovered in 1984 and is the most robust genomic abnormality observed in about 20% of neuroblastoma [26]. Gene copies can range from four to over 1000, and *MYCN* gene amplification is significantly associated with rapid tumor growth and disease progression [27].

As well as CNAs, the gene expression of neuroblastoma cells was investigated by microarray technology. Gene expression profiling was found significantly different between localized and metastatic tumors. Oberthuer et al. [28, 29] have identified a 144-gene signature associated with tumor aggressiveness and poor patients' outcome. Moreover, a 59-gene signature has been also found associated with patient's risk although neither 144- nor 59-gene signatures are currently used as prognostic markers [30]. Recently, we have looked for the global gene expression between localized and metastatic tumors. This difference was calculated for each gene and called as transcription instability (TIN), and we generated a TIN-index that is significantly higher in metastatic tumor in respect of the localized one. Our study shows that gene expression is highly deregulated in advanced tumors [submitted manuscript].

5. One, two, multistep: the tumorigenesis of neuroblastoma

The tumorigenesis of neuroblastoma is still unclear. Neuroblastoma shows a great biological and genetics heterogeneity, suggesting that more than one gene is involved in the tumor initiation and progression. Neuroblastoma stroma-poor shows great potential of growth and rapidly forms metastases distally from primary tumor, indicating that gene mutations increase the tumor cell invasion capacity. On the contrary, ganglioneuroblastoma has low aggressiveness, indicating that not all gene mutations are critical for tumor growth and invasion. Ganglioneuroblastoma is composed by malignant neuroblasts and Schwannian stromal cells; the latter, possibly, are playing a tumor suppression activity by regulating the tumor microenvironment. Indeed, several observations report a complex cross-talk between neuroblastoma cells and Schwannian stroma cells, manly mediated by cytokines [31, 32]. Lastly, neuroblastoma cells of clinical stage 4S still are a fascinating problem, because this metastatic tumor can regress spontaneously. To explain disease regression of stage 4S tumor, it has been proposed that neuroblastoma cells are delayed to achieve the complete cell differentiation before the birth of patient, but the cell maturation is completed within the first year of patient's age [33].

Knudson and Meadows [34] have suggested the presence of a recessive NB gene to explain the behavior of stage 4S tumor, a model resembling the recessive RB gene discovered in retinoblastoma. Since chromosome 1p36 region has been found deleted in more than 40% of cases, this region was a candidate locus to contain NB-suppressor gene [35]. Indeed, if one NB gene would be located in the deleted chromosome 1p36 region, the two-hit model should be fit in the carcinogenesis of neuroblastoma. Unfortunately, linkage analysis of neuroblastoma pedigrees has not revealed NB-genes in the 1p36 region.

Recently, animal models that recapitulate the genesis of neuroblastoma are produced in mouse and in zebrafish. *MYCN* human oncogene has been overexpressed in transgenic mouse, demonstrating that tumor growth is under *MYCN* control. Similarly, neuroblastoma can grow in mouse overexpressing *ALK* or *LIN28*. In zebrafish model, the overexpression of *MYCN* gene blocks the development of sympathoadrenal precursor toward the chromaffin-like cells, inducing the formation of neuroblastoma cells in the interrenal gland. Neuroblastoma tumor growing in both mouse and zebrafish resembles human neuroblastoma in many of aspects such as cell morphology [36]. Zebrafish has been also employed to study the embryonic development of NCC. These cells can be easily identified by the expression of *SOX10* (Sry-box 10) and *Crestin* genes that are expressed in migratory NCC. So, the precise and detailed analysis of NCC development during physiological embryonic life of zebrafish can greatly help to generate new models for the study of neuroblastoma tumorigenesis.

Finally, since several chromosome regions are affected in neuroblastoma tumor, it is reasonable to think that numerous genes are impaired giving a sort of multifactorial or multistep damage to the normal cells [37]. Loss of chromosome 1p36 region, 3p, 4p, 9p 11q 14q together gain of 1q, 2p24, 12p, 17q, mutations of *ALK* and receptor tyrosine kinase (*AXL*) gene, and telomerase reverse transcriptase (TERT) re-arrangements may be seen as mutational steps, leading to the transformation of normal neural crest cell to neuroblastoma cell.

In this contest, the role of gene mutation seems not sufficient to transform the normal cell into neuroblastoma, at least for all Neuroblastic Tumors because the frequency of gene mutation in neuroblastoma, as well as other pediatric cancer, is dramatically lower than mutations observed in adult cancer. On the other hand, few genes can have critical damaging mutations that are dangerous for the pathways in which genes work, suggesting an oligogenic mechanism of neuroblastoma tumorigenesis [38].

6. Chromosome instability and neuroblastoma

The low number of mutations in neuroblastoma suggests that abnormalities in gene sequencing play a role in some but not in all neuroblastoma. The more aggressive tumors are belonging to patients over one year of age with metastatic disease; these patients with stage 4 disease have a median age of onset between four and five years. Differently from infants' patients, tumor cells of stage 4 patients over one year of age have several nonrandom structural CNAs. Others and we have suggested that tumor cells of these patients accumulate chromosome damages in a time-dependent manner [39, 40]. As consequence, this suggests a multistep manner of neuroblastoma development and it is reasonable to think that several alterations such as single gene mutation, gene deletion, gene amplification, gene rearrangement, and gross chromosome aberrations participate in the neuroblastoma tumorigenesis. This hypothesis is also supported by the discovery of chromothripsis, a catastrophic defect mainly occurring in chromosome 5 that damages almost all chromosome regions [41]. More recently, I suggested that chromosomal instability (CIN) plays a crucial role in the neuroblastoma development [42]. CIN is a feature of most cancers and can be caused by abnormal mitosis, failure in the microtubule and centrosome dynamics, or spindle apparatus, abnormal control of double-strand break repair, telomere maintenance, and abnormal telomere function. Several genes are involved in the mentioned mechanisms, and so they can be considered CIN-related genes. Carter et al. [43] have proposed two CIN: CIN25 and CIN70 (the number shows the number of genes considered in the signature) expression signatures that were used to predict survival in lung adenocarcinoma, medulloblastoma, breast cancer, lymphoma and other tumors. Unfortunately, neither CIN25 nor CIN70 was a good prognostic marker in neuroblastoma. **Table 1** shows some genes included in the CIN signatures together with genes that are involved in the mitotic control and that can contribute to CIN after their deregulation. The complexity of CIN is shown by the presence of at least two CIN: the whole chromosome instability (W-CIN) characterized by additional entire chromosome and the segmental chromosome instability (S-CIN) that shows chromosome structural changes such as deletion, amplification and rearrangements.

In neuroblastoma, we often found W-CIN in localized stage 1 and 2 tumors, while both W-CIN and S-CIN are detectable in tumors of stage 3, 4 and 4S. How W-CIN and S-CIN can contribute to the tumorigenesis is still unclear. A mathematical model [44] indicates that abnormal numerical whole chromosome number occurs very early in stage 4S (**Figure 3**). Additional whole chromosome aberration is followed by segmental chromosome damage in stage 4 tumors. So, we can argue that W-CIN is beginning in stage 4S and W-CIN together with S-CIN is present in stage 4.

Gene	Locus	OMIM	Function
ATRX	Xq21.1	300032	Associated with pericentromeric heterochromatin during interphase and mitosis; ATRX protein is also associated with chromosomes during mitosis
AURKA	20q13.2	603072	Induction of centrosome duplication-distribution abnormalities and aneuploidy
AURKB	17p13.1	604970	Direct interaction between CENPA and AURKA
BRRN1	2q11.2	602332	Involved in interphase and mitotic condensation
BUB1	2q13	602452	Protects centromeric cohesion during mitosis throughout SGO1
CNAP1	20q11.22	609689	Human rootletin (CROCC) bound CNAP1 at the proximal end of centrioles and formed the bridge between two centrioles
CDCA8	1p34.3	609977	CDCA8 interacts with AURKB and survivin (BIRC5)
CDC2	10q21.2	116940	Coordinates spindle assembly with the cell cycle during mitosis through phosphorylation of RCC
CDC20	1q34.2	603618	CDC20 together with HCDH1 active APC during mitosis and G1
CCNB1	5q13.2	123836	CCNB1 with p34 (cdc2) (CDK1) form a mitosis-promoting factor
CENPE	4q24	117143	Associates with kinetochores
ECT2	3q26.31	600586	ECT2 is localized in central spindle at anaphase and promotes local activation of RhoA GTPase
ESPL1	12q13.13	604143	Loss of sister chromatid cohesion activity
FOXM1	12p13.33	602341	Regulates expression of cell cycle proteins
H2AFX	11q23.3	601772	Involved in chromatin conformation
MAD2L1	4q27	601467	Induction of chromosome instability by overexpression of the mitotic checkpoint gene Mad2
NEK2	1q32.3	604043	Overexpression of active NEK2 induces a splitting of centrosomes
KIF4A	Xq13.1	300521	In HeLa cells, KIF4 interacted directly during spindle midzone formation
PTTG1	5q33.3	604147	PTTG1 appeared to be an anaphase-promoting complex
PRC1	15q26.1	603484	In HeLa cells, PRC1 together KIF4 interacted directly during spindle midzone formation
TOP2A	17q21.2	126430	Involved in chromosome segregation
TPX2	20q11.21	605917	Involved in microtubule organization during mitosis and normal spindle morphology
TTK	6q14.1	604092	Regulator of genetic stability and spindle apparatus

In the Table are listed genes participating in the CIN. The chromosome locus, OMIM code and function are reported for each gene. Some genes such as *AURKAB, BUB1, CNAP1* and *CDCA8* cooperate with other genes in the control of genetics stability and mitotic checkpoint (derived from Refs. [43, 45]).

Table 1. Genes involved in CIN.

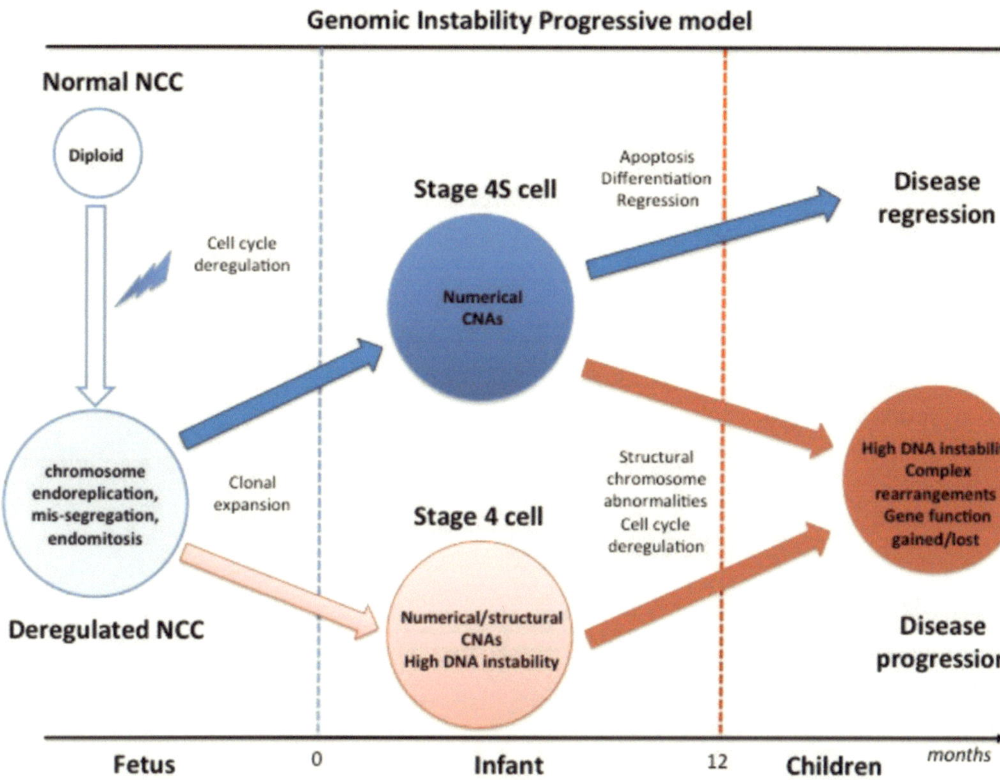

Figure 3. Model of genomic instability in neuroblastoma. The model suggests that tumor of stage 4S and 4 originates from NCC by numerical copy number abnormalities (CNAs) for stage 4S and numerical together with structural CNAs for stage 4. After infant life, only tumors with high genomic instability either stage 4S or stage 4 develop, contributing to disease progression [44].

As underlined before, Neuroblastic Tumors show biological and morphological heterogeneous features. It is possible that genotype-phenotype aspects reflect diverse road of the genesis of this tumor in which different genes are involved with different critical damages. This scenario makes the study of neuroblastoma tumorigenesis very complex.

7. Conclusion

Today, we have a huge amount of biological and clinical data of neuroblastoma. We know genome mutations and gene expression abnormality occurring in neuroblastoma cells. However, all data are referring to the tumor cells at onset of the disease and in same cases at relapse. Up to now, we have no information about the tumorigenesis of the tumor. The initial phases of tumor growth and progression are very important for the diagnosis and treatment of neuroblastoma. Very few mutations are present in this pediatric cancer, and the mutational two-step or multistep models do not completely fitting with the neuroblastoma tumorigenesis. We develop a mathematical models to explain the genesis of this tumor. Moreover, we have several information about the chromosome damage and chromothripsis, suggesting that CIN plays a crucial role in neuroblastoma tumorigenesis. Some animal models seem to recapitulate the development of the tumor, focusing our attention to few crucial genes. However, we are still in the dark zone and the origin and development of neuroblastoma remains unsolved.

Acknowledgements

The work was supported by Italian Neuroblastoma Foundation (Fondazione Italiana per la Lotta al Neuroblastoma).

Author details

Gian Paolo Tonini

Address all correspondence to: gp.tonini@irpcds.org

Neuroblastoma Laboratory, Pediatric Research Institute, Città della Speranza, Padua, Italy

References

[1] Esposito MR, Aveic S, Seydel A, Tonini GP. Neuroblastoma treatment in the post-genomic era. Journal of Biomedical Science. 2017;**24**(1):14

[2] Schramm A, Koster J, Assenov Y, Althoff K, Peifer M, Mahlow E, Odersky A, Beisser D, Ernst C, Henssen AG, et al. Mutational dynamics between primary and relapse neuroblastomas. Nature Genetics. 2015;**47**(8):872-877

[3] Tonini GP, Nakagawara A, Berthold F. Towards a turning point of neuroblastoma therapy. Cancer Letters. 2012;**326**:128-134

[4] Haupt R, Garaventa A, Gambini C, Parodi S, Cangemi G, Casale F, Viscardi E, Bianchi M, Prete A, Jenkner A, et al. Improved survival of children with neuroblastoma between 1979 and 2005: A report of the Italian Neuroblastoma Registry. Journal of Clinical Oncology: Official Journal of the American Society of Clinical Oncology. 2010;**28**(14):2331-2338

[5] Nakagawara A, Ohira M. Comprehensive genomics linking between neural development and cancer: Neuroblastoma as a model. Cancer Letters. 2004;**204**(2):213-224

[6] De Preter K, Vandesompele J, Heimann P, Yigit N, Beckman S, Schramm A, Eggert A, Stallings RL, Benoit Y, Renard M, et al. Human fetal neuroblast and neuroblastoma transcriptome analysis confirms neuroblast origin and highlights neuroblastoma candidate genes. Genome Biology. 2006;**7**(9):R84

[7] Luksch R, Castellani MR, Collini P, De Bernardi B, Conte M, Gambini C, Gandola L, Garaventa A, Biasoni D, Podda M, et al. Neuroblastoma (peripheral neuroblastic tumours). Critical Reviews in Oncology/Hematology. 2016;**107**:163-181

[8] Matthay KK, Maris JM, Schleiermacher G, Nakagawara A, Mackall CL, Diller L, Weiss WA. Neuroblastoma. Nature Reviews Disease Primers. 2016;**2**:16078

[9] Shimada H, Ambros IM, Dehner LP, Hata J, Joshi VV, Roald B, Stram DO, Gerbing RB, Lukens JN, Matthay KK, et al. The International Neuroblastoma Pathology Classification (the Shimada system). Cancer. 1999;**86**(2):364-372

[10] Tonini GP. Neuroblastoma: A multiple biological disease. European Journal of Cancer. 1993;**29A**(6):802-804

[11] Maris JM, Hogarty MD, Bagatell R, Cohn SL. Neuroblastoma. Lancet. 2007;**369**:2106-2120

[12] Ikeda Y, Lister J, Bouton JM, Buyukpamukcu M. Congenital neuroblastoma, neuroblastoma in situ, and the normal fetal development of the adrenal. Journal of Pediatric Surgery. 1981;**16**(4 Suppl 1):636-644

[13] Gigliotti AR, Di Cataldo A, Sorrentino S, Parodi S, Rizzo A, Buffa P, Granata C, Sementa AR, Fagnani AM, Provenzi M, et al. Neuroblastoma in the newborn. A study of the Italian Neuroblastoma Registry. European Journal of Cancer. 2009;**45**(18):3220-3227

[14] Longo L, Panza E, Schena F, Seri M, Devoto M, Romeo G, Bini C, Pappalardo G, Tonini GP, Perri P. Genetic predisposition to familial neuroblastoma: Identification of two novel genomic regions at 2p and 12p. Human Heredity. 2007;**63**(3-4):205-211

[15] Mosse YP, Laudenslager M, Longo L, Cole KA, Wood A, Attiyeh EF, Laquaglia MJ, Sennett R, Lynch JE, Perri P, et al. Identification of ALK as a major familial neuroblastoma predisposition gene. Nature. 2008;**455**(7215):930-935

[16] Stanton BR, Parada LF. The N-myc proto-oncogene: Developmental expression and in vivo site-directed mutagenesis. Brain Pathology. 1992;**2**(1):71-83

[17] Iwahara T, Fujimoto J, Wen D, Cupples R, Bucay N, Arakawa T, Mori S, Ratzkin B, Yamamoto T. Molecular characterization of ALK, a receptor tyrosine kinase expressed specifically in the nervous system. Oncogene. 1997;**14**(4):439-449

[18] Bosse KR, Diskin SJ, Cole KA, Wood AC, Schnepp RW, Norris G, Nguyen le B, Jagannathan J, Laquaglia M, Winter C, et al. Common variation at BARD1 results in the expression of an oncogenic isoform that influences neuroblastoma susceptibility and oncogenicity. Cancer Research. 2012;**72**(8):2068-2078

[19] Oldridge DA, Wood AC, Weichert-Leahey N, Crimmins I, Sussman R, Winter C, McDaniel LD, Diamond M, Hart LS, Zhu S, et al. Genetic predisposition to neuroblastoma mediated by a LMO1 super-enhancer polymorphism. Nature. 2015;**528**(7582):418-421

[20] Schnepp RW, Khurana P, Attiyeh EF, Raman P, Chodosh SE, Oldridge DA, Gagliardi ME, Conkrite KL, Asgharzadeh S, Seeger RC, et al. A LIN28B-RAN-AURKA signaling network promotes neuroblastoma tumorigenesis. Cancer Cell. 2015;**28**(5):599-609

[21] Schleiermacher G, Michon J, Ribeiro A, Pierron G, Mosseri V, Rubie H, Munzer C, Bénard J, Auger N, Combaret V, et al. Segmental chromosomal alterations lead to a higher risk of relapse in infants with MYCN-non-amplified localised unresectable/disseminated neuroblastoma (a SIOPEN collaborative study). British Journal of Cancer. 2011;**105**:1940-1948

[22] Scaruffi P, Coco S, Cifuentes F, Albino D, Nair M, Defferrari R, Mazzocco K, Tonini GP. Identification and characterization of DNA imbalances in neuroblastoma by high-resolution oligonucleotide array comparative genomic hybridization. Cancer Genetics and Cytogenetics. 2007;**177**(1):20-29

[23] Stigliani S, Coco S, Moretti S, Oberthuer A, Fischer M, Theissen J, Gallo F, Garavent A, Berthold F, Bonassi S, et al. High genomic instability predicts survival in metastatic high-risk neuroblastoma. Neoplasia. 2012;**14**:823-832

[24] Tonini GP, Romani M. Genetic and epigenetic alterations in neuroblastoma. Cancer Letters. 2003;**197**(1-2):69-73

[25] Janoueix-Lerosey I, Schleiermacher G, Michels E, Mosseri V, Ribeiro A, Lequin D, Vermeulen J, Couturier J, Peuchmaur M, Valent A, et al. Overall genomic pattern is a predictor of outcome in neuroblastoma. Journal of Clinical Oncology: Official Journal of the American Society of Clinical Oncology. 2009;**27**:1026-1033

[26] Schwab M, Alitalo K, Klempnauer KH, Varmus HE, Bishop JM, Gilbert F, Brodeur G, Goldstein M, Trent J. Amplified DNA with limited homology to myc cellular oncogene is shared by human neuroblastoma cell lines and a neuroblastoma tumour. Nature. 1983;**305**(5931):245-248

[27] Brodeur GM, Seeger RC, Schwab M, Varmus HE, Bishop JM. Amplification of N-myc in untreated human neuroblastomas correlates with advanced disease stage. Science. 1984;**224**(4653):1121-1124

[28] Oberthuer A, Berthold F, Warnat P, Hero B, Kahlert Y, Spitz R, Ernestus K, Konig R, Haas S, Eils R, et al. Customized oligonucleotide microarray gene expression-based classification of neuroblastoma patients outperforms current clinical risk stratification. Journal of Clinical Oncology: Official Journal of the American Society of Clinical Oncology. 2006;**24**(31):5070-5078

[29] Oberthuer A, Hero B, Berthold F, Juraeva D, Faldum A, Kahlert Y, Asgharzadeh S, Seeger R, Scaruffi P, Tonini GP, et al. Prognostic impact of gene expression-based classification for neuroblastoma. Journal of Clinical Oncology: Official Journal of the American Society of Clinical Oncology. 2010;**28**(21):3506-3515

[30] Vermeulen J, De Preter K, Naranjo A, Vercruysse L, Van Roy N, Hellemans J, Swerts K, Bravo S, Scaruffi P, Tonini GP, et al. Predicting outcomes for children with neuroblastoma using a multigene-expression signature: A retrospective SIOPEN/COG/GPOH study. The Lancet Oncology. 2009;**10**(7):663-671

[31] Del Grosso F, Coco S, Scaruffi P, Stigliani S, Valdora F, Benelli R, Salvi S, Boccardo S, Truini M, Croce M, et al. Role of CXCL13-CXCR5 crosstalk between malignant

neuroblastoma cells and Schwannian stromal cells in neuroblastic tumors. Molecular Cancer Research: MCR. 2011;**9**(7):815-823

[32] Gross N, Meier R. Chemokines in neuroectodermal cancers: The crucial growth signal from the soil. Seminars in Cancer Biology. 2009;**19**(2):103-110

[33] Pritchard J, Hickman JA. Why does stage 4S neuroblastoma regress spontaneously? Lancet. 1994;**344**(8926):869-870

[34] Knudson AG Jr, Meadows AT. Sounding board. Regression of neuroblastoma IV-S: A genetic hypothesis. The New England Journal of Medicine. 1980;**302**(22):1254-1256

[35] Lo Cunsolo C, Iolascon A, Cavazzana A, Cusano R, Strigini P, Mazzocco K, Giordani L, Massimo L, De Bernardi B, Conte M, et al. Neuroblastoma in two siblings supports the role of 1p36 deletion in tumor development. Cancer Genetics and Cytogenetics. 1999;**109**(2):126-130

[36] Corallo D, Candiani S, Ori M, Aveic S, Tonini GP. The zebrafish as a model for studying neuroblastoma. Cancer Cell International. 2016;**16**:82

[37] Tonini GP. Neuroblastoma: The result of multistep transformation? Stem Cells. 1993;**11**(4):276-282

[38] Perri P, Longo L, Cusano R, McConville CM, Rees SA, Devoto M, Conte M, Ferrara GB, Seri M, Romeo G, et al. Weak linkage at 4p16 to predisposition for human neuroblastoma. Oncogene. 2002;**21**(54):8356-8360

[39] Schleiermacher G, Janoueix-Lerosey I, Ribeiro A, Klijanienko J, Couturier J, Pierron G, Mosseri V, Valent A, Auger N, Plantaz D, et al. Accumulation of segmental alterations determines progression in neuroblastoma. Journal of Clinical Oncology: Official Journal of the American Society of Clinical Oncology. 2010;**28**(19):3122-3130

[40] Coco S, Theissen J, Scaruffi P, Stigliani S, Moretti S, Oberthuer A, Valdora F, Fischer M, Gallo F, Hero B, et al. Age-dependent accumulation of genomic aberrations and deregulation of cell cycle and telomerase genes in metastatic neuroblastoma. Journal international du cancer [International Journal of Cancer]. 2012;**131**:1591-1600

[41] Molenaar JJ, Koster J, Zwijnenburg DA, van Sluis P, Valentijn LJ, van der Ploeg I, Hamdi M, van Nes J, Westerman BA, van Arkel J, et al. Sequencing of neuroblastoma identifies chromothripsis and defects in neuritogenesis genes. Nature. 2012;**483**(7391):589-593

[42] Tonini GP. Growth, progression and chromosome instability of neuroblastoma: A new scenario of tumorigenesis? BMC Cancer. 2017;**17**(1):20

[43] Carter SL, Eklund AC, Kohane IS, Harris LN, Szallasi Z. A signature of chromosomal instability inferred from gene expression profiles predicts clinical outcome in multiple human cancers. Nature Genetics. 2006;**38**(9):1043-1048

[44] Masecchia S, Coco S, Barla A, Verri A, Tonini GP. Genome instability model of metastatic neuroblastoma tumorigenesis by a dictionary learning algorithm. BMC Medical Genomics. 2015;**8**:57

[45] Schvartzman JM, Sotillo R, Benezra R. Mitotic chromosomal instability and cancer: Mouse modelling of the human disease. Nature Reviews Cancer. 2010;**10**(2):102-115

Chapter 3

Anatomic Origin and Molecular Genetics in Neuroblastoma

Murat Tosun, Hamit Selim Karabekir,
Mehmet Ozan Durmaz, Harun Muayad Said,
Yasemin Soysal and Nuket Gocmen Mas

Additional information is available at the end of the chapter

http://dx.doi.org/10.5772/intechopen.69568

Abstract

Neuroblastoma is considered as the most common extracranial solid tumor occurring during childhood, but takes place rarely after the age of 10 years. The tumors are considered as embryonal tumors that result from the fetal or early postnatal life development and are formed from neural crest-derived cells, and their origination is from the early nerve cells which are called as neuroblasts of sympathetic nervous system. Being heterogeneous in their biological, genetic, and morphological characteristics, tumors which are distinct from other solid tumors due to their biological heterogeneity result in the clinical pattern changes from spontaneous regression to a highly aggressive metastatic disease. Neuroblastoma tumorigenesis is regulated by Myc oncogene, leading to aggressive tumor subset. Many epigenetic factors play crucial role in the disease induction and development, while regulatory effect and outcome result in epigenetic patterns distinguishing neuroectoderm, neural crest, and more mature neural states. Neuroblastoma patients' clinical management is based on prognostic categories subtracted from studies correlating outcome and clinico-biological variables. Neuroblastoma anatomic boundaries include primarily autonomic nervous system besides other rare locations. Neuroblastoma molecular pathogenesis classifies the tumor according to the different clinical behaviors that are important for the improvement of the patients outcome and overall survival according to the different therapy modalities applied.

Keywords: neuroblastoma, anatomy, clinic, genetics

1. Introduction

Neuroblastoma is the most common extracranial solid tumor in childhood; moreover, it is very rare after age of 10 years. They are regarded as embryonal tumors developed during fetal or

INTECH
open science | open minds

© 2017 The Author(s). Licensee InTech. This chapter is distributed under the terms of the Creative Commons Attribution License (http://creativecommons.org/licenses/by/3.0), which permits unrestricted use, distribution, and reproduction in any medium, provided the original work is properly cited.

early postnatal life and arise from the immature or dedifferentiated neural crest-derived cells. It is important to understand that they originate from the early nerve cells which are called as neuroblasts of the sympathetic nervous system, so they can be found anywhere along this system.

The system includes sympathetic trunk and ganglia, adrenal medulla, and also an aggregation of cells called as paraganglion [1].

2. The autonomic nervous system

The autonomic nervous system (ANS) is a part of peripheral nervous system, and under the control of the central nervous system, it governs many involuntary processes of the body such as heart rate, vascular tone, glandular activity, digestive motility, and others. It has two main contents as the sympathetic (thoracolumbar—from T1 to L2) and parasympathetic (craniosacral—from S2 to S4 and parasympathetic cranial nerves) systems. These two main systems contain both preganglionic and postganglionic neurons which are governed by hypothalamus. Posterior part of the hypothalamus is related to the sympathetic system [1–4]. Sympathetic nervous system starts to develop from the neural crest cells, and anterior part of the neural tube of the thoracic region migrates on either side of the spinal cord, toward the region behind the dorsal aorta about week 5 of embryogenesis. Some of them leave neural tube in order to arrange along the motor root [5, 6]. Mammalian neural crest cells are multipotent cells and originate from ectoderm. It has been accepted as the fourth layer of embryo for some researcher, because of their contribution to the cellular diversity in vertebrates. During embryological development, neural crest cells migrate from neural tube and differentiate into different structures including adrenomedullary cells and sympathetic neurons in adrenergic system. The ganglia cells of the thoracic region migrate during 5th week of development. Neural crest cells forming sympathetic ganglia also migrate both cranially and caudally and extend these trunks into cervical and pelvic regions. The migration and localization of neural crest cells are controlled by bone morphogenetic proteins (BMP) secreted by dorsal aorta [7–9].

3. Gross anatomy of sympathetic trunk and ganglia

The sympathetic ganglia together with the suprarenal (adrenal) medulla and chromaffin cells of paraganglia are derived from the sympathoadrenal linage cells. From the suprarenal medulla, these cells differentiate into a number of types consisting of small and intermediate-sized neuroblasts and sympathoblasts and larger, initial rounded phechromocytoblasts. Large cells harboring pale nuclei might be the progenitors of chromaffin cells. These cells secrete either adrenaline (epinephrine) or noradrenaline (norepinephrine), while the intermediate-sized neuroblasts differentiate into the typical multipolar postganglionic symphatic neurons, and secrete only noradrenaline while paraganglia, situated near, on the surface of, or embedded in, the capsules of the ganglia of the sympathetic chain, or in some of the large autonomic plexuses which are cell masses called paraganglion [10–12].

The sympathetic system consists of two ganglionated trunks together with their branches, plexuses, and subsidiary ganglia, while the sympathetic ganglia include sympathetic trunk cell aggregations in the autonomic plexuses and intermediate ganglia while the plexuses contain dispersed preganglionic cells (**Figure 1**).

Trunks ganglia correspond numerically to the dorsal spinal roots ganglia, while adjoining ganglia may fuse in man and there are rarely more than 22 or 23 and sometimes fewer. Subsidiary ganglia in the major autonomic plexuses (e.g., coeliac, superior mesenteric ganglia, etc.) are trunks ganglia derivates [13–20].

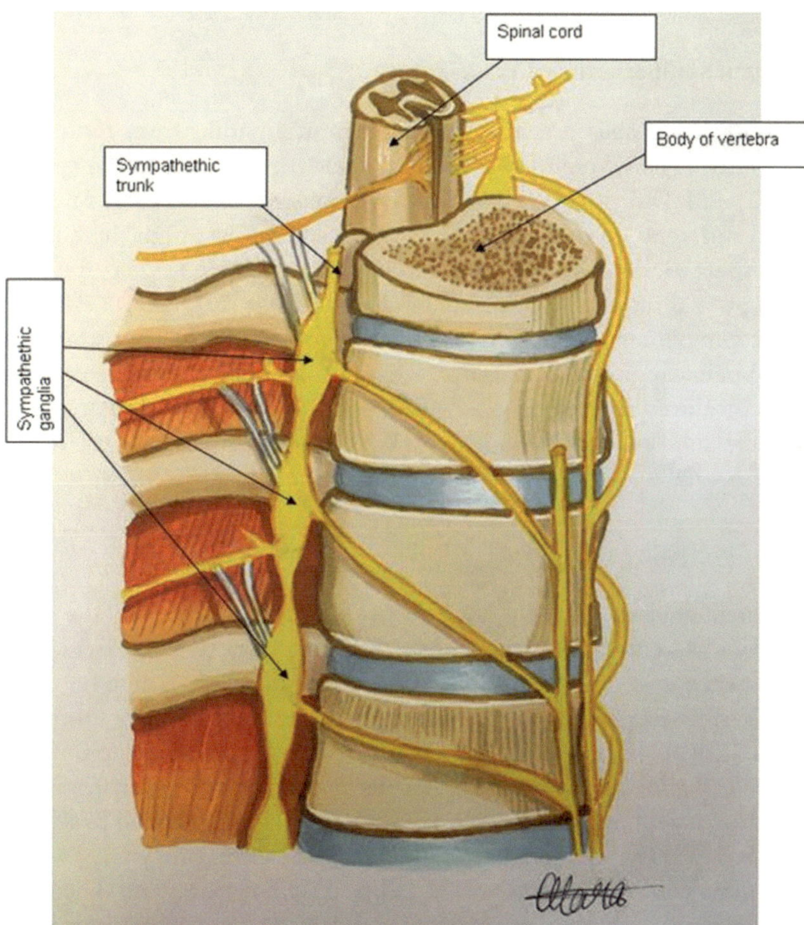

Figure 1. Components of the sympathetic trunk. Redrawn from Wolf-Heidegger's Atlas of Human Anatomy.

The sympathetic trunk is positioned just laterally to the vertebral bodies for the entire vertebral column length and interacts with the spinal nerves anterior rami via rami communicantes. The sympathetic trunk allows the sympathetic nervous system including the preganglionic fibers to ascend to spinal levels superior to T1 and descend to spinal levels inferior to L2/3. The sympathetic trunk ganglion returns to the spinal nerve of preganglionic origin via gray ramus comminicans, while the higher end was continuing via the carotid canal forming at the end a plexus located at the internal carotid artery and on the other hand the lower parts move before the coccyx and at this position it merges with the other ganglion impar basal structures. Paravertebral ganglia are sympathetic ganglia along the length of the sympathetic trunk which is a sympathetic nervous system and also a basal part of the autonomic nervous system. It enables nerve fibers to extend toward the spinal nerves located at a superior position as well as inferior position to those they were emanated from. We have here also to mention that various nerves like a high percentage of the splanchnic nerves emerge directly from this trunks [14–20].

3.1. Embryology of sympathetic trunk

Mammalian neural crest cells are multipotent cells originating from the ectoderm. They represent the fourth layer of embryo because of their contribution to the cellular diversity in vertebrates [21–23]. During embryological development, neural crest cells migrate from neural tube and differentiate into different structures including both the adrenomedullary cells and the sympathetic neurons in the adrenergic system (**Table 1**). Also, the thoracic region ganglia cells migrate at the end of 5th week of development [22]. Neural crest cells forming the sympathetic ganglia also migrate both cranially and caudally and extend these trunks into cervical and pelvic regions. Bone morphogenetic proteins (BMP) secreted by dorsal aorta norepinephrine produced by notochord control neural crest cell migration and localization, while at the same time and molecular level, Wnt/β-catenin-related Gbx2 homeobox gene deactivation is essential for the neural crest development [22, 23].

3.2. Histology of sympathetic ganglia

The nervous system anatomically divides into two parts which are both the central and the peripheral nervous systems, and at the same time, it was functionally divided into somatic and autonomic nervous systems including sympathetic and parasympathetic subdivisions. All the nervous system was built from two main structures, namely the neurons and glial cells in intercellular matrix. Neurons differ in their type being bipolar, pseudounipolar or motor, while three types of glial cells can be seen in the neural matrix including all of the astrocytes, oligodendroglia and microglia [24, 25]. All neurons have two main processes, axon and dendrites, and two of them form an extremely dense connecting network and where all the processes make synapses with each other [24, 25]. The signals from central neurons are transported from presynaptic membrane to postsynaptic membrane via neurotransmitters such as serotonin, dopamine, acetylcholine, epinephrine (E) [adrenalin (A)] and norepinephrine (NE) [noradrenaline (NA)] [24, 25]. One of the main differences between neuron functions

Neural Crest	
Cranial Neural Crest Cell	Trunk Neural Crest Cell
- Diencephalic Neural Crest Cell - Mesencephalic Neural Crest Cell - Rhomboencephalic Neural Crest Cell - Cardiac Neural Crest Cell	- Chromaffin cells in adrenal medula - Dorsal Root Ganglia - Epidermal pigment cells (Melanocytes) - Satellite Glial Cells - Tooth Papilae - Corneal endothelium and stroma - Sympathetic neurons - Vagal Neural Crest Cells - Calcitonin Secreting Cells - Carotid body type I Cells - Multipolar neurons in sympathetic ganglion

Table 1. Structures formed from the neural crest cell differentiation.

is which kind of neurotransmitters being secreted for signal transmission in synaptic space. In adrenergic neurons, E and NE are named as catecholamines, while dopamine is the main neurotransmitter synthesized from tyrosine NE and serves as a transmitter between axons and effectors in autonomic nervous system [24]. Neurons using NE as a neurotransmitter are adrenergic neurons. Epinephrine is secreted by some both the central nervous system cells and the endocrine chromaffin cells in the adrenal medulla [24, 25].

3.3. Genetics and clinical characteristics

It has been shown in Ref. [26] that both the dicer and miRNAs are required for the survival of neural crest-derived tissues by preventing apoptosis during differentiation because the dicer was essential for the differentiation process related to the neural crest cells survival, while neuronal crest needs specific hdac1 function during its development as shown in a series of zebrafish experiment [27]. In the trunk region, the ventrally migrating neural crest cells move through the somitic mesenchyme in a segmented pattern, presumably setting the basis for the sensory and sympathetic ganglia metameric organization along the anterior-posterior axis later in development [28].

When grafting experiments were performed, a specific migratory behavior of the cells was observed which was under the control of the cellular microenvironment endowed by both the surrounding mesenchymal cells and the extra cellular matrix (ECM). Also, the posterior sclerotome which represents a nonpermissive tissues generative barriers for the movement of the neuronal crest cells is formed together with the perinotochordal region and, transiently, the tissue located below the dorsolateral ectoderm [29–31]. Neural crest cells reorganize as they migrate; formation of iterated, discrete sympathetic ganglia is not the direct result of patterned crest cell migration through the somites, and the chain formation is a common configuration adopted by migrating cells in the developing nervous system [32]. Also it has been shown in [33] that the parasympathetic neurons originate from nerve-associated peripheral glial progenitors besides that the development of noradrenergic neurons in the hindbrain medulla and in the sympathetic nervous system depends on retinoic acid signaling in addition to the fact that the mount Blanc mutation disrupts the development of noradrenergic centers in the CNS and of sympathetic ganglia [34, 35].

4. Adrenal medulla

The adrenal glands also develop from neural crest ectoderm and intermediate mesoderm. While the medulla originated from neural crest cells migrating from sympathetic ganglion, adrenal cortex develops from intermediate mesoderm. During the 5th week of development, proliferating mesothelium-derived cells infiltrate the retroperitoneal mesenchyme at the cranial end of the mesonephros and give rise to the primitive adrenal cortex. Further, a second layer of proliferated cells surrounds the primitive cortex and, as a consequence, forms the future adult adrenal cortex. At the 7th week of development, the mesothelial cells are invaded at its medial region by neural crest-derived chromaffinoblast cells. These cells differentiate into two kinds of chromaffin cells of the adrenal medulla which renders homologous to a diffuse sympathetic ganglion without postganglionic processes, leading to complete development of the adrenal gland at the 4th month of age. Further, the fetal cortex regresses and disappears within the 1st year of life with replacement by the definitive cortex [36–45].

The cells migrating from the neural tube compose two chains of sympathetic ganglia at both sides of the vertebral column. One of them is lateral vertebral sympathetic chain that occurs from the interconnecting ganglia by longitudinal nerve fibers and the other ones: superior cervical ganglion, the middle cervical ganglion and the inferior cervical ganglion; lumbosacral region of the sympathetic ganglia occurs from the neuroblast migration and extends from thoracic region. Some of the sympathetic neuroblasts migrate further anteriorly to form preaortic ganglia as celiac and mesenteric plexuses, the visceral ganglia of the Auerbach myenteric plexus and in the Meissner submucous plexus [41–45].

4.1. Gross anatomy of adrenal medulla

For the position of the adrenal glands, they are both positioned on the two sides of the body located at the retroperitoneum slightly elevated and at medial position from the kidneys. It is a characteristic of the human adrenal glands that their shape differs according to its position, possessing a pyramidal shape for the right adrenal gland versus a larger and semilunar shape for the left adrenal glands. Adrenal gland size also differs depending on the age of the subject but in average they are 5.3 cm in size and 7–10 g in weight. The glands are yellowish in

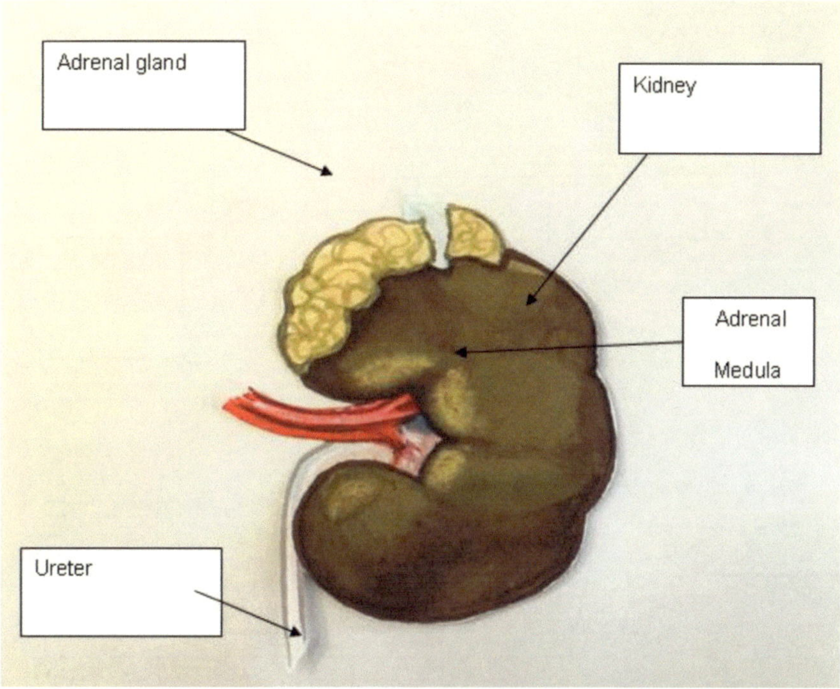

Figure 2. The components from the adrenal medulla. Redrawn from Wolf-Heidegger's Atlas of Human Anatomy.

color and surrounded by a fatty capsule and lie within the renal fascia which also surrounds the kidneys, while a weak wall of connective tissue separates the glands from the kidneys (**Figure 2**) [41–45].

The adrenal glands are positioned directly below the diaphragm and attached to the diaphragm crura by the renal fascia. The adrenal gland is consisted of two distinct parts, the outer adrenal cortex and the inner medulla, each with a unique function, but both produce hormones. The adrenal medulla is at the center of each adrenal gland and is surrounded by the adrenal cortex. The chromaffin cells of the medulla are the body's main source of the catecholamine's adrenaline and noradrenalin, released by the medulla (**Figure 3**) [41–45].

The adrenal medulla is driven by the sympathetic nervous system via preganglionic fibers originating in the thoracic spinal cord, from vertebrae T5–T11. Because it is innervated by preganglionic nerve fibers, the adrenal medulla can be considered as a specialized sympathetic ganglion. Unlike other sympathetic ganglia, however, the adrenal medulla lacks distinct synapses and releases its secretions directly into the blood [41–45]. The sympathetic nervous system through the preganglionic fibers that are originated from the thoracic spinal cord at the vertebrae T5–T11 controls the adrenal medulla, which can be considered as a specialized sympathetic ganglion due to its strengthening via the preganglionic nerve fibers. One of the characteristics of the adrenal medulla was that it differs from the sympathetic ganglion that is latching of independent synapses and its secretions are released into the blood by a direct manner [41–45]. These hormones are released by the adrenal medulla, which contains a dense

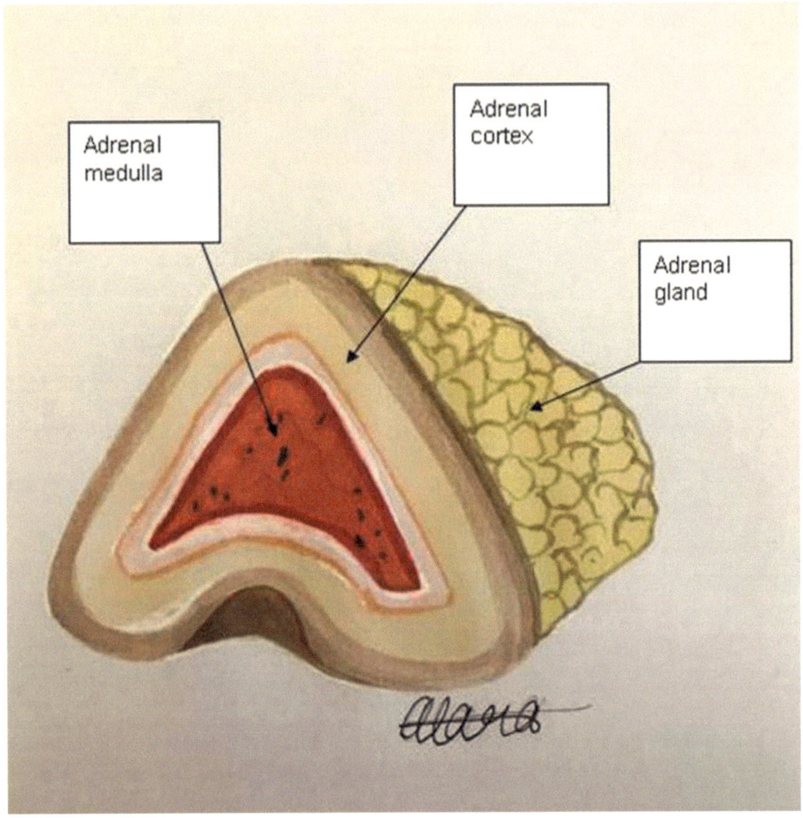

Figure 3. The components from the adrenal gland. Redrawn from Wolf-Heidegger's Atlas of Human Anatomy.

network of blood vessels. Adrenaline and noradrenaline act at adrenoreceptors throughout the body, leading to increase both the circulating blood pressure and heart beat speed also known as heart rate. There is also a phenomenon called "flight response" where both adrenalin and noradrenalin are responsible for it and this phenomenon of increasing the speed of breathing, heartbeat, and blood pressure is due to the increased blood vessel contraction in the different parts of the body [46, 47]. Catecholamines are produced in chromaffin cells in the medulla of the adrenal gland, from tyrosine, a nonessential amino acid either derived from food or produced from phenylalanine in the liver. Suprarenal medulla is composed of chromaffin cell column groups separated by wide venous sinusoids, while single and small groups of neurons occur in the medulla. Tyrosine hydroxylase converts tyrosine to L-DOPA during the initial step of catecholamine synthesis with further conversion of L-DOPA to dopamine prior to its conversion into noradrenaline. On the other hand, the enzyme phenylethanolamine N-methyltransferase (PNMT) converts noradrenaline into epinephrine and becomes stored in cytosolic granules.

Tyrosine hydroxylase and PNMT levels play an important regulative role in the catecholamines synthesis in a way that when their level increases they affect the adrenal cortex glucocorticoids that in turn stimulate the catecholamine synthesis, where the sympathetic nervous system via its activation stimulates the catecholamine release. Also, the adrenal gland medulla is innervated by the sympathetic nervous system splanchnic nerves, where as a consequence the stimulation of the cell membrane calcium channels opening evokes the release of the catecholamines from the storage granules [41–45, 48–52]. Adrenal gland's medulla and para-aortic body tumors can cause excessive adrenaline and noradrenaline secretion, leading to palpitation attacks, excessive sweating, pallor, hypertension, headaches and retinitis and renal vascular changes as a consequence of a long persistence of the tumor [41–45].

4.2. Embryology of the adrenal gland

The adrenal glands develop from neural crest ectoderm and intermediate mesoderm. While the medulla originated from neural crest cells migrating from sympathetic ganglion, adrenal cortex was developed from the intermediate mesoderm [42]. During the 5th week of development, proliferating mesothelium-derived cells infiltrate the retroperitoneal mesenchyme at the cranial end of the mesonephros and give rise to the primitive adrenal cortex [23–25]. A second proliferation of these cells surrounds the primitive cortex and forms the future adult adrenal cortex. At the 7th week of development, neural crest-derived chromaffinoblast cells invade the mesothelial cells at its medial region [24]. These cells differentiate into chromaffin cells of the adrenal medulla. The adrenal medulla is homologous to a diffuse sympathetic ganglion without postganglionic processes [24]. At the 4th month of age, the adrenal gland is fully developed. The fetal cortex regresses and disappears within the 1st year of life and is replaced by the definitive cortex. During adrenal gland development, some transcription factors such as Wnt4 and Wnt1 have very important regularity functions [53].

4.3. Histology of adrenal gland

Histologically, the adrenal glands (**Figure 4**) have two main structures, one of which is the cortex including three substructures (**Figure 3**) and medulla (**Figure 5**). The cortex cover with capsule contains collagen and elastic fibers and has three layers, and each has different functions: the outermost, zona glomerulosa, the middle, zona fasciculata and the innermost layer, zona reticularis. Although zona glomerulosa cells produce aldosterone, zona fasciculate cells mainly produce cortisol, while zona reticularis cells synthesize androgen. Both zona fasciculata and reticularis are stimulated by adrenocorticotropic hormone (ACTH), but zona glomerulosa is primarily stimulated by angiotensin II that stimulates both zona glomerulosa and proliferation and aldosterone synthesis [24, 25]. The adrenal medulla is located in the adrenal gland center and contains the chromaffin cells, which are modified sympathetic postganglionic neurons derived from neural crest, and forms epithelioid cords surrounded by fenestrated capillaries [24]. Chromaffin cell cytoplasm contains membrane-bounded dense granules containing chromogranins, one class of catecholamine epinephrine and norepinephrine and a little dopamine. Two kinds of chromaffin cells exist in the adrenal medulla, 80% of which produce epinephrine and 20% of which produce norepinephrine that is stored in granules with a dense eccentric core, while epinephrine contains granules that are smaller and occupy less dense central core, whereas all circulating epinephrine produced by adrenal medulla, norepinephrine produces both adrenal medulla and postganglionic sympathetic neurons, but we have to mention here that adrenal cortex cells do not store their steroid hormones in granules [24, 25].

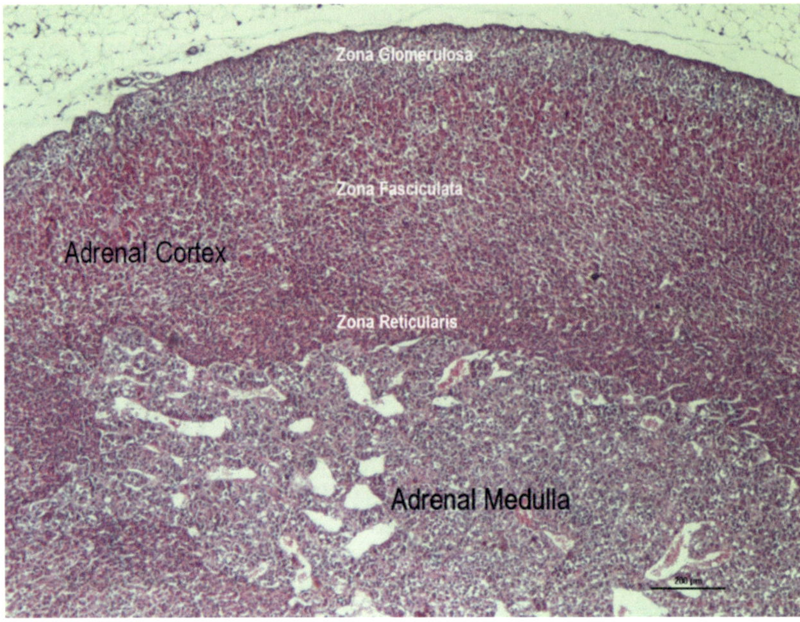

Figure 4. General microscopic view of the adrenal gland. Hematoxylin-eosin staining. 400× (image recorded and edited by Murat TOSUN MD PhD).

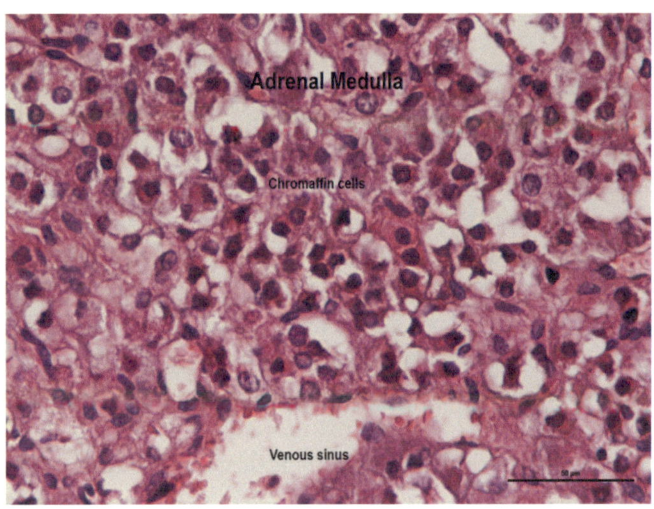

Figure 5. Microscopic view of the adrenal medulla. Hematoxylin-eosin. 400× (image recorded and edited by Murat TOSUN MD PhD).

The adrenal medulla is composed of groups and columns of chromaffin cells (phaeochromocytes) separated by wide venous sinusoids and supported by a network of reticular fibers. Chromaffin cells bear the name as a result of their response to the use of dichromate fixative during the fixation process. Structurally and functionally, they are comparable to the postganglionic sympathetic neurons being at the same time a member of the neuroendocrine system.

Since they are derived from the neuronal crest, they produce, store before release and release different hormones into the venous sinusoids which are catecholamines, noradrenalin (or as mentioned in other references norepinephrines) or adrenaline. The synthesis, storage and release of these hormones are under the control of the sympathetic nervous system precisely by the sympathetic neurons where the preganglion and their sympathetic neurons are shown as a single appearance or as a small group located at the medulla. When the noradrenaline-secreting cells are rarely present, they possess bigger sized granules having a dense eccentric kernel [5, 6, 54–56]. Normally, cells differ in their hormone secretion manner. While some cells secret only hormone, others are secreting two hormones. Catecholamines together with enkephalins represent opiate like proteins that are under certain conditions pached by the chromogranin proteins. The cells that are formed here are shown as large cells possessing a large nuclei with a cytoplasmic region that is faintly granular and basophilic ahead the venous sinusoids and in a single-lined alignment. The sympathetic axon terminals are forming synapses together with the chromaffin cells where these synapses are positioned locations opposite and distant to the sinusoids. These sinusoids in turn are arranged via a branched construct of cells called the fenestrated endothelium and elapse to both the central medullar vein and the Hilary suprarenal vein, while according to the knowledge available until now the suprarenal medulla presence and function do not represent a necessity for life activities [57, 58].

Further, we have here to address that the scientific community should concentrate their research efforts to study the different aspects of the adrenal medulla since the information available about it is restricted and the availability of it can help to unravel many unknown points about the development of this disease.

4.4. Genetic and clinical investigations of adrenal medulla

For the establishment of genetic parameters of neuroblastomas, continuous scientific efforts were necessary [59]. In molecular and genetic analysis, different pathology-related findings were possible. One research group was able to prove experimentally that activated ALK collaborates with MYCN during neuroblastoma pathogenesis where they used the Zebrafish model that was able to help them proving that neuroblastomas arise in MYCN expressing transgenic Zebrafish and showing the MYCN-induced loss of sympathoadrenal cells; the absence of expression of early sympathoadrenal markers was absent in MYCN transgenic embryos during early development; MYCN expression causes sympathoadrenal cell loss and the role of the activated ALK in the disease onset acceleration and increases the penetrance of MYCN-induced neuroblastoma [60]. Experimentally, the direct role of dopamine in the generation and/or expansion of mitochondrial DNA deletions in dopaminergic neurons was proven unraveling more knowledge about the Parkinson's disease pathogenesis, showing here the mitochondrial DNA deletions accumulation role and representing the missing link between aging and Parkinson's disease, while the catecholaminergic adrenal medulla is the preferential location of mitochondrial DNA deletions [61]. Also in another experimental setup, gene expression profiling helped to identify eleven DNA repair genes downregulated during mouse neural crest cell migration process [62]. Radiotherapy, chemotherapy and surgery are only suitable for neuroblastomas treatment but MIBG (metaiodobenzylguanidine) application, and nuclear medicine has a dual function aiding in diagnosis as well as its function as a treatment modality, but immunological methods like the application of a monoclonal antibody and proved to be more effective and promising when applied at early stages [63–65].

5. Paraganglion

5.1. Gross anatomy, embryology and histology of the paraganglion

Paraganglia are extrasuprarenal chromaffin tissue aggregations that distribute (near to/within) the automatic nervous system. This type of paraganglia cells also occurs in the sympathetic ganglia of various viscera as well as in variety of retroperitoneal and mediastinal sites; all of these cells synthesize and store catecholamines and are derived from the neural crest, and their function is defined by their position. Being a remainder source of neuroendocrine secretion, intraneuronal cells are functioning as interneurons. In suprarenal medulla, chemical stimuli are responsible for catecholamine release, while the role of the neuronal stimuli is neglectable regarding to this functional detail. Within the fetus, the extrasuprarenal chromaffin tissue is representing the main repository of catecholamine where within this regard the suprarenal medulla plays no role due to the fact of being immature.

However, many paraganglia are well vascularized and their secretory cells are usually close to one or more fenestrated capillaries. Most like the suprarenal medullary chromaffin cells, they have a sympathetic innervation and thereby act as endocrine organs [1]. Para-aortic bodies and coccygeal body (glomus coccygeum) are paraganglia which include chromaffin cells and produce adrenaline and noradrenaline. Para-aortic bodies place on lateral side of abdominal aorta and usually united anterior to it by a horizontal mass immediately above the inferior mesenteric artery [13].

5.2. Coccygeal body

The coccygeal glomus (coccygeal gland or body also it is referred as the Luschka's coccygeal body by others) represents a vestigial structure situated either in front of or immediately below the coccyx tip that is situated near the ganglion impar in the pelvis in addition to another position near the median sacral artery termination [66]. Its diameter is 2.5 mm and has an irregular oval shape; several smaller nodules are found around or near the main mass and consist of irregular masses of round or polyhedral cells or epithelioid cells, forming a group around a dilated sinusoidal capillary vessel [66–68].

Each cell includes a large round or oval nucleus and the protoplasm surrounding the nucleus which is clear, and not stained when chromic salts are applied; therefore, it is not considered as a part of chromaffin system, the system which includes cells stained by chromic salts and consists of renal medulla, paraganglia and para-aortic bodies [66–68]. Clinically, the coccygeal body looks like a glomus tumor, thereby causing problems in the diagnosis that can lead to misinterpretations [69–71].

Paraganglia are extrasuprarenal aggregations of chromaffin tissue, distributed near to or within the autonomic nervous system. This type of cells also occurs in the sympathetic ganglia of various viscera and in a variety of retroperitoneal and mediastinal sites. All of these cells are derived from the neural crest, and all of them synthesize and store catecholamines. Also, their function depends on the way and site they are positioned; several cells role is functioning as interneurons, while in other cases, there are cells existing that are functioning in another manner within this context by acting as a source for the neuroendocrine secretion. In the coccygeal bodies, chemical inducers are responsible of the paraganglionic release of catecholamines. The period of the paraganglion existence in human is different, while their regulating factors and mechanisms are still not completely understood, and a population of them keep present until adulthood mostly as a microscopic paraganglia with its later degeneration [36–40].

6. Para-aortic bodies

The para-aortic bodies are chromaffin tissue condensations found closely to the aortic autonomic plexuses and lumbar sympathetic chains. In the fetus, they are at the largest size but later become relatively smaller in childhood and disappear at the beginning of the adulthood. Mostly, their presence of existence is as a pair of bodies positioned within intermesenteric, inferior mesenteric and hypogastric plexus anterolaterally to the aorta. They can be elevated at the celiac plexus or bounded below at the hypogastric plexus of the pelvis, or can be nearby the sympathetic ganglia of the lumbar chain. Scattered cells, which persist into adulthood, may rarely be the chromaffin tissue tumor development sites (phaeochromocytoma); these scattered cells are much more commonly found arising from the suprarenal medulla cells. The wide variation in the persistent para-aortic body tissue site accounts for the range of locations of such tumors [54, 55, 72].

7. Experimental treatment of neuroblastoma cells: *in vitro*

During a series of experiments conducted that aimed to evaluate cytotoxic effects of melatonin (MLT) which is an endogen hormone and 13-*cis* retinoic acid (13-*cis*-RA) also named as isotretinoin a vitamin A analogue on neuroblastoma SH-SY5Y cell line by our research group [73]. We found that treatment of neuroblastoma cells with melatonin resulted into a cytotoxic effect in a way where in cell culture the cells were exposed to different doses of MLT and 13-*cis*-RA for either 24 or 48 h. While the viabilities were estimated with MTT cell viability assay test, apoptotic indexes were calculated after staining with TUNEL-based apoptosis determination. We observed the effective cytotoxic potential on neuroblastoma cell line which MLT l poses which was higher than the one 13-*cis*-RA. At the same time, when MLT and 13-*cis*-RA were combined, the obtained effect was potentiated. On the other hand, it was found that the effect of 13-*cis*-RA individually was very slight. Results gathered from the current study have indicated that MLT exhibited neurotoxic effect on SH-SY5Y neuroblastoma cell line and this effect was potentiated by 13-*cis*-RA.

As a consequence, we believe that administration of these agents in neuroblastoma patient treatment may contribute to obtain outcomes that bear potential for the design of innovative treatment modalities, leading to the successful treatment of this type of diseases, with taking in account the necessity of *in vivo* studies based on these results that clearly determine the dose range necessary. It is expected that the results of them can improve the currently applied treatment modalities applied against neuroblastomas to be more successful.

8. Conclusions

Neuroblastoma is the most common extracranial solid tumor occurring during childhood till the age of 10 when it might occur rarely. Many epigenetic factors play a crucial role in the disease induction and development of neuroblastoma, while the regulatory effect and outcome resulting into epigenetic patterns is well known but needs further study. Different research efforts were made by various research groups to study this type of disease from the different levels, where some results like neuroblastoma treatment with melatonin was one positive example, while the study of the adrenal medulla needs to be more intensified by the scientific community since the understanding of its different regulatory aspects can be one target for the optimization of the treatment methods applied against this disease.

Acknowledgements

The authors would like to thank the Dokuz Eylul University and the Afyon Kocatepe University for their kind support. Also, we would like to thank Ms. Alara Karabekir for the graphic design. Finally, we also would like to thank Assoc. Prof. Dr Nilüfer Yonguc from the Dokuz Eylül University and Mr Ali Ege Mas from the Near Eastern University, Cyprus, for technical support during the different stages of the research.

Author details

Murat Tosun[1*], Hamit Selim Karabekir[2], Mehmet Ozan Durmaz[3], Harun Muayad Said[4], Yasemin Soysal[4] and Nuket Gocmen Mas[5]

*Address all correspondence to: murat_tosun@yahoo.com

1 Department of Histology and Embryology, Faculty of Medicine, Afyon Kocatepe University, Afyonkarahisar, Turkey

2 Department of Neurosurgery, Faculty of Medicine, Dokuz Eylul University, Izmir, Turkey

3 Department of Neurosurgery, Bozyaka Education and Research Hospital, Health Science University, Izmir, Turkey

4 Department of Molecular Medicine, Graduate Institute of Health Science, Dokuz Eylul University, Izmir, Turkey

5 Department of Anatomy, Faculty of Medicine, Dokuz Eylul University, Izmir, Turkey

References

[1] Standring S. Gray's Anatomy. 39th ed. Elsevier, Churchill Livingstone, London 2005. pp. 419-430

[2] McCorry LK. Physiology of the autonomic nervous system. American Journal of Pharmaceutical Education. 2007;**71**(4):78

[3] Shields RW Jr. Functional anatomy of the autonomic nervous system. Journal of Clinical Neurophysiology. 1993;**10**(1):2-13

[4] Amann JF, Constantinescu GM. The anatomy of the visceral and autonomic nervous systems. Seminars in Veterinary Medicine and Surgery (Small Animal). 1990;**5**(1):4-11

[5] Selleck MA, Bronner-Fraser M. Origins of the avian neural crest: The role of neural plate-epidermal interactions. Development. 1995;**121**(2):525-538

[6] Thorogood P. Review of developmental and evolutionary aspects of the neural crest. Trends in Neurosciences. 1989;**12**:38-39

[7] Bhatt S, Diaz R, Trainor PA. Signals and switches in mammalian neural crest cell differentiation. Cold Spring Harbor Perspectives in Biology. 2013;**5**(2):a008326. DOI: 10.1101/cshperspect.a008326

[8] Motohashi T, Watanabe N, Nishioka M, et al. Gene array analysis of neural crest cells identifies transcription factors necessary for direct conversion of embryonic fibroblasts into neural crest cells. Biology Open. 2016;**5**(3):311-322. DOI: 10.1242/bio.015735

[9] Simões-Costa M, Bronner ME. Establishing neural crest identity: A gene regulatory recipe. Development. 2015;**142**(2):242-257. DOI: 10.1242/dev.105445

[10] Morrison SF, Cao WH. Different adrenal sympathetic preganglionic neurons regulate epinephrine and norepinephrine secretion. American Journal of Physiology. Regulatory, Integrative and Comparative Physiology. 2000;**279**(5):R1763-R1775

[11] Rubin RP, Miele E. A study of the differential secretion of epinephrine and norepinephrine from the perfused cat adrenal gland. Journal of Pharmacology and Experimental Therapeutics. 1968;**164**(1):115-121

[12] Standring S. Gray's Anatomy. 39th ed. Elsevir Churchill Livingstone, London; 2005. pp. 181-182, 254-255

[13] Standring S. Gray's Anatomy. 38th ed. Churchill Livingstone, London; 1995. pp. 1905-1906

[14] Mader SS. Human Biology. New York: McGraw-Hill; 2000. ISBN: 0-07-290584-0; ISBN: 0-07-117940-2

[15] Pritchard TE, Alloway D. Medical Neuroscience. FL, United States: Hayes Barton Press; 1999. ISBN: 978-1-59377-200 0. Available from: https://books.google.com/books/about/Medical_neuroscience.html?id=m7Y80PcFHtsC

[16] Butler AB, Hodos W. Comparative Vertebrate Neuroanatomy: Evolution and Adaptation. Hoboken, NJ, US: Wiley-Blackwell; 2005. ISBN: 978-0-471-21005-4

[17] Hall JE, Guyton AC. Textbook of Medical Physiology. 11th ed. St. Louis, MO: Elsevier Saunders; 2006. ISBN: 0-7216-0240-1

[18] Warrell DA, Cox TM, Firth JD. The Oxford Textbook of Medicine. 5th ed. Philadelphia, Pennsylvania, US: Oxford University Press; 2010

[19] Greenstein B, Greenstein A. Color Atlas of Neuroscience: Neuroanatomy and Neurophysiology. Stuttgart, New York: Thieme; 2002. ISBN: 9783131081711

[20] Moore KL, Agur AMR. Essential Clinical Anatomy. 2nd ed. Philadelphia, Pennsylvania, US: Lippincott Williams & Wilkins. 2002. p. 199. ISBN: 978-0-7817-5940-3

[21] Gilbert SF. The cranial neural crest. In: Developmental Biology. 6th ed. Sinauer Associates. Bookshelf ID: NBK10065, Oxford, UK: Oxford University Press, ISBN-10: 0-87893-243-7

[22] Moore KL, Persaud TVN, Torchia MG. Development of suprarenal glands. In: The Developing Human: Clinically Oriented Embryology. 9th ed. Elsevier Saunders, Philadelphia, 2012

[23] Carlson BM. Neural crest. In: Human Embryology and Developmental Biology. 5th ed. Carlson BM. Elsevier Saunders, Philadelphia, 2014

[24] Kiezenbaum AL, Tres LL. Adrenal gland. In: Histology and Cell: An Introduction to Pathology. 3rd ed. Elsevier Saunders, Philadelphia, 2012

[25] Abrahamsohn I, Dos Santos MF, Tenario Zorn TM. Endocrine glands. In: Basic Histology (Text & Atlas). 11th ed. McGraw Hill: NY, USA 2005

[26] Zehir A, Hua LL, Maska EL, Morikawa Y, Cserjesi P. Dicer is required for survival of differentiating neural crest cells. Developmental Biology. 2010;**340**(2):459-467. DOI: 10.1016/j.ydbio.2010.01.039

[27] Ignatius MS, Unal Eroglu A, Malireddy S, Gallagher G, Nambiar RM, Henion PD. Distinct functional and temporal requirements for zebrafish Hdac1 during neural crest-derived craniofacial and peripheral neuron development. PLoS One. 2013;**8**(5):e63218. DOI: 10.1371/journal.pone.0063218

[28] Krull CE. Segmental organization of neural crest migration. Mechanisms of Development. 2001;**105**:37-45

[29] Bronner-Fraser M, Stern C. Effects of mesodermal tissues on avian neural crest cell migration. Developmental Biology. 1991;**143**:213-217

[30] Pettway Z, Guillory G, Bronner-Fraser M. Absence of neural crest cells from the region surrounding implanted notochords in situ. Developmental Biology. 1990;**142**:335-345

[31] Erickson CA, Duong TD, Tosney KW. Descriptive and experimental analysis of the dispersion of neural crest cells along the dorsolateral path and their entry into ectoderm in the chick embryo. Developmental Biology. 1992;**151**(1):251-272

[32] Kasemeier-Kulesa JC, Kulesa PM, Lefcort F. Imaging neural crest cell dynamics during formation of dorsal root ganglia and sympathetic ganglia. Development. 2005;**132**(2):235-245. DOI: 10.1242/dev.01553

[33] Dyachuk V, Furlan A, Shahidi MK, Giovenco M, Kaukua N, Konstantinidou C, Pachnis V, Memic F, Marklund U, Müller T, Birchmeier C, Fried K, Ernfors P, Adameyko I. Neurodevelopment. Parasympathetic neurons originate from nerve-associated peripheral glial progenitors. Science. 2014;**345**(6192):82-87. DOI: 10.1126/science.1253281

[34] Holzschuh J, Barrallo-Gimeno A, Ettl AK, Durr K, Knapik EW, Driever W. Noradrenergic neurons in the zebrafish hindbrain are induced by retinoic acid and require tfap2a for expression of the neurotransmitter phenotype. Development. 2003;**130**(23):5741-5754

[35] Holzschuh J, Hauptmann G, Driever W. Genetic analysis of the roles of Hh, FGF8, and nodal signaling during catecholaminergic system development in the zebrafish brain. Journal of Neuroscience. 2003;**23**(13):55. DOI: 10.1242/dev.00816

[36] Zhang S, Su Y, Gao J, Zhang C, Tanaka H. A potential inhibitory function of draxin in regulating mouse trunk neural crest migration. In Vitro Cellular & Developmental Biology-Animal. 2017;**53**(1):43-53. DOI: 10.1007/s11626-016-0079-0

[37] Ezin M, Barembaum M, Bronner ME. Stage-dependent plasticity of the anterior neural folds to form neural crest. Differentiation. 2014;**88**(2-3):42-50. DOI: 10.1016/j.diff.2014.09.003

[38] Serralbo O, Marcelle C. Migrating cells mediate long-range WNT signaling. Development. 2014;**141**(10):2057-2063. DOI: 10.1242/dev.107656

[39] Ridenour DA, McLennan R, Teddy JM, Semerad CL, Haug JS, Kulesa PM. The neural crest cell cycle is related to phases of migration in the head. Development. 2014;**141**(5):1095-1103. DOI: 10.1242/dev.098855

[40] Shyamala K, Yanduri S, Girish HC, Murgod S. Neural crest: The fourth germ layer. Journal of Oral and Maxillofacial Pathology. 2015;**19**(2):221-229. DOI: 10.4103/0973-029X.164536

[41] Thomas P. Endocrine Gland Development and Disease. Burlington: Elsevier Science. Academic Press, Cambridge, Massachusetts, US, 2013. p. 241. ISBN: 9780123914545

[42] Moore KL, Dalley AF, Agur AM. Clinically Oriented Anatomy. 7th ed. Philadelphia, Pennsylvania, US: Lippincott Williams & Wilkins; 2013. pp. 294-298. ISBN: 978-1-4511-8447-1

[43] Kay SM, Flageole H. Adrenal Glands. Medscape, 2015. http://emedicine.medscape.com/article/940347-overview [Accessed: August 1, 2015]

[44] Dunn, R. B.; Kudrath, W.; Passo, S.S.; Wilson, L.B. (2011). "10". Kaplan USMLE Step 1 Physiology Lecture Notes. pp. 263-289.endothelial cells: roles of PPAR alpha and NF-kappaB.Vascul Pharmacol. **48**(2-3): 76-84

[45] Sapru HN, Siegel A. Essential Neuroscience. Hagerstown, MD: Lippincott Williams & Wilkins; 2007. ISBN: 0-7817-9121-9

[46] Goldstein DS, Kopin IJ. Evolution of concepts of stress. Stress. 2007;**10**(2):109-120. DOI: 10.1080/10253890701288935

[47] Weems CF, Silverman WK. An integrative model of control: Implications for understanding emotion regulation and dysregulation in childhood anxiety. Journal of Affective Disorders. 2006;**91**(2-3):113-124. DOI: 10.1016/j.jad.2006.01.009

[48] Melmed S, Polonsky KS, Larsen PR, Kronenberg HM. Williams Textbook of Endocrinology. 12th ed. London, UK: Saunders; 2011. ISBN: 978-1437703245

[49] Whitehead SA, Nussey S. Endocrinology: An Integrated Approach. Oxford: BIOS; 2001. p. 122. ISBN: 1-85996-252-1

[50] Colledge NR, Walker BR, Ralston SH, editors. Davidson's Principles and Practice of Medicine. Illustrated by Robert Britton. 21st ed. Edinburgh: Churchill Livingstone/ Elsevier; 2010. pp. 768-778. ISBN: 978-0-7020-3085-7

[51] Henry G, Alan JF, Daniel R. Psychology. 6th ed. NY, US: W. W. Norton & Company; 2004. ISBN: 0-393-97767-6

[52] García AG, García de Diego AM, Gandía L, Borges R, García Sancho J. Calcium signaling and exocytosis in adrenal chromaffin cells. Physiological Reviews. 2006;**86**(4):1093-1131. DOI: 10.1152/physrev.00039.2005. PMID: 17015485

[53] Schoenwolf GC, Belyl SB, Brauer PR, Francis-West PH. Development of suprarenal gland. In: Larsen's Human Embryology. 4th ed. Churchill Livingstone, 2008, eBook ISBN: 9780323286190, eBook ISBN: 9781437700909, eBook ISBN: 9780323240116; 2009

[54] Coupland RE, Kent C, Kent SE. Normal function of extra-adrenal chromaffin tissues in the young rabbit and guinea-pig. Journal of Endocrinology. 1982;**92**(3):433-442

[55] Galan-Rodriguez B, del-Marco A, Flores JA, Ramiro-Fuentes S, Gonzalez-Aparicio R, Tunez I, Tasset I, Fernandez-Espejo E. Grafts of extra-adrenal chromaffin cells as aggregates show better survival rate and regenerative effects on Parkinsonian rats than dispersed cell grafts. Neurobiology of Disease. 2008;**29**(3):529-542. DOI: 10.1016/j.nbd.2007.11.009

[56] Unsicker K, Zwarg U, Habura O. Electron microscopic evidence for the formation of synapses and synaptoid contacts in adrenal medullary grafts. Brain Research. 1977;**120**(3):533-539

[57] Hoshi N, Hitomi J, Kusakabe T, Fukuda T, Hirota M, Suzuki T. Distinct morphological and immunohistochemical features and different growth rates among four human neuroblastomas heterotransplanted into nude mice. Medical Molecular Morphology. 2008;**41**(3):151-159. DOI: 10.1007/s00795-008-0407-x

[58] Hirose T, Kannuki S, Nishida K, Matsumoto K, Sano T, Hizawa K. Anaplastic ganglioglioma of the brain stem demonstrating active neurosecretory features of neoplastic neuronal cells. Acta Neuropathologica. 1992;**83**(4):365-370

[59] Bilke S, Chen QR, Westerman F, Schwab M, Catchpoole D, Khan J. Inferring a tumor progression model for neuroblastoma from genomic data. Journal of Clinical Oncology. 2005;**23**(29):7322-7331. DOI: 10.1200/JCO.2005.03.2821. [Epub: September 6, 2005]

[60] Zhu S, Lee JS, Guo F, Shin J, Perez-Atayde AR, Kutok JL, Rodig SJ, Neuberg DS, Helman D, Feng H, Stewart RA, Wang W, George RE, Kanki JP, Look AT. Activated ALK collaborates with MYCN in neuroblastoma pathogenesis. Cancer Cell. 2012;**21**(3):362-373. DOI: 10.1016/j.ccr.2012.02.010

[61] Neuhaus JF, Baris OR, Hess S, Moser N, Schröder H, Chinta SJ, Andersen JK, Kloppenburg P, Wiesner RJ. Catecholamine metabolism drives generation of mitochondrial DNA deletions in dopaminergic neurons. Brain. 2014;**137**(Pt 2):354-365. DOI: 10.1093/brain/awt291. [Epub: October 24, 2013]

[62] Albino D, Brizzolara A, Moretti S, Falugi C, Mirisola V, Scaruffi P, Di Candia M, Truini M, Coco S, Bonassi S, Tonini GP. Gene expression profiling identifies eleven DNA repair genes down-regulated during mouse neural crest cell migration. International Journal of Developmental Biology. 2011;**55**(1):65-72. DOI: 10.1387/ijdb.092970da

[63] Cheung NV, Kushner BH, Kramer K. Monoclonal antibody based therapy of neuroblastoma. Hematology/Oncology Clinics of North America. 2001;**15**(5):853-866

[64] Saarinen UM, Coccia PF, Gerson SL, et al. Eradication of neuroblastoma cells in vitro by monoclonal antibody and human complement: Method for purging autologous bone marrow. Cancer Research. 1985;**45**(11):5969-5975

[65] Conti A, Maestroni GJ, Cosentino M, Frigo GM, Lecchini S, Marino F, Bombelli R, Ferrari M, Brivio F, Roselli MG, Lissoni P. Evidence for a neuroimmunomodulatory and a hematopoietic role of the Luschka's coccygeal body. Neuroendocrinology Letters. 2000;**21**(5):391-403

[66] Rahemtullah A, Szyfelbein K, Zembowicz A. Glomus coccygeum: Report of a case and review of the literature. American Journal of Dermatopathology. 2005;**27**(6):497-499

[67] Kim HS, Yang SH, Park HJ, Park HB, Cho HS. Glomus tumor as a cause of coccydynia. Skeletal Radiology. 2013;**42**(10):1471-1473. DOI: 10.1007/s00256-013-1654-z. [Epub: June 4, 2013]

[68] Gatalica Z, Wang L, Lucio ET, Miettinen M. Glomus coccygeum in surgical pathology specimens: Small troublemaker. Archives of Pathology and Laboratory Medicine. 1999;**123**(10):905-908

[69] Albrecht S, Zbieranowski I. Incidental glomus coccygeum. When a normal structure looks like a tumor. American Journal of Surgical Pathology. 1990;**14**(10):922-924

[70] Santos LD, Chow C, Kennerson AR. Glomus coccygeum may mimic glomus tumour. Pathology. 2002;**34**(4):339-343

[71] Vergote I, Amant F, Berteloot P, Van Gramberen M. Laparoscopic lower para-aortic staging lymphadenectomy in stage IB2, II, and III cervical cancer. International Journal of Gynecological Cancer. 2002;**12**(1):22-26

[72] Tosun M, Soysal Y, Mas NG, Karabekir HS. Comparison of the effects of 13-cis retinoic acid and melatonin on the viabilities of SH-SY5Y neuroblastoma cell line. Journal of Korean Neurosurgical Society. 2015;**57**(3):147-151. DOI: 10.3340/jkns.2015.57.3.147

[73] Köpf-Maier P. Wolf-Heidegger's Atlas of Human Anatomy. 6th ed. Karger (Berlin) Karger AG; Basel, 2005. ISBN: 978-3-8055-7667-3

Chapter 4

Target Therapy in Neuroblastoma

Tamer Hassan, Mohamed Badr, Usama El Safy,
Mervat Hesham, Laila Sherief, Mohamed Beshir,
Manar Fathy, Mohamed Al Malky and
Marwa Zakaria

Additional information is available at the end of the chapter

http://dx.doi.org/10.5772/intechopen.70328

Abstract

Neuroblastoma is an embryonal malignancy that originates in the sympathetic nervous system. It is the most common solid tumor in infants and the most frequent extracranial solid tumor in children. Neuroblastoma accounts for 10% of childhood malignancies with 75% occurring in children <4 years. Stage, age, clinical and tumor genomic features are the principal criteria for determining treatment policy. Treatment modalities traditionally employed in the management of neuroblastoma are surgery, chemotherapy, and radiotherapy. Intensive multimodal treatment in patients with neuroblastoma has resulted in improved survival rates. However, there is a considerable percentage of patients with refractory and relapsed disease. Targeted therapy for neuroblastoma involves treatment aimed at molecular targets that have a unique expression in this childhood cancer. A large number of molecular targets have been identified for the treatment of high-risk and relapsed neuroblastoma. Treatment in this way aims at providing a more selective way to treat the disease and decreasing toxicities associated with the conventional treatment regimen.

Keywords: neuroblastoma, target, therapy, refractory, relapse

1. Introduction

Neuroblastoma, originating in neural crest cells, can occur anywhere along the sympathetic nerve chain. By far the most common location for a primary tumor is the adrenal gland. In its most primitive form, the histology of neuroblastoma is marked by poorly differentiated small, round blue cells. At an intermediate stage of maturation, there is differentiation

INTECH
open science | open minds

© 2017 The Author(s). Licensee InTech. This chapter is distributed under the terms of the Creative Commons Attribution License (http://creativecommons.org/licenses/by/3.0), which permits unrestricted use, distribution, and reproduction in any medium, provided the original work is properly cited.

toward ganglion cells. Tumors composed of a mixture of neuroblasts and mature ganglion cells are classified as ganglioneuroblastomas. At the most differentiated end of the spectrum is ganglioneuroma, a benign tumor composed entirely of mature ganglion cells, neuritis, and Schwann cell [1].

At diagnosis, 65% of patients have disseminated disease, most commonly spreading to the bone. Disseminated disease is typically manifested as fever and bone pain. Additionally, neuroblastoma is associated with a paraneoplastic syndrome of opsoclonus-myoclonus ("dancing eyes and feet syndrome") [2].

Treatment modalities traditionally employed in the management of neuroblastoma are surgery, chemotherapy, and radiotherapy. Recently immunotherapy has been established as an important component of advanced neuroblastoma treatment. Intensive multimodal treatment strategies improved the survival in children with neuroblastoma. However, issues related to treatment refractoriness and late effects as well as disease recurrence remain significant challenges [3].

Multiple therapeutic targets have been developed to offer an advantage of treating neuroblastoma in a more selective way to maximize the treatment efficacy and minimize its toxicity [3].

1.1. Neuroblastoma staging systems

Several staging systems have been used to classify disease extent. The International Neuroblastoma Staging System (INSS), which is based on clinical and surgical evaluations, was developed by consensus of major pediatric oncology groups (POGs) in the United States, Europe, and Japan. The INSS differentiates between INSS stages 1, 2A, 2B, 3, 4, and 4S, based on surgical excision, lymph node involvement, and metastatic sites [4].

Because the INSS is a surgically based staging system, the stage for patients with locoregional disease can vary based on degree of surgical resection. Noteworthy, patients with localized disease who will not undergo surgery cannot be adequately staged. For these reasons, the International Neuroblastoma Risk Group (INRG) Task Force developed a new pretreatment staging system in 2005 based on clinical criteria and specific image-defined risk factors. Required imaging modalities include CT or MRI, as well as MIBG scintigraphy. The International Neuroblastoma Risk Group Staging System (INRGSS) differentiates between L1, L2, M, and MS stages. The INRGSS differs from the INSS in that the INRGSS is based on preoperative imaging characteristics and not on surgical resection. The age for the INRGSS MS stage is set at 547 days (18 months) compared with 12 months in the INSS 4S stage (**Table 1**) [5].

1.2. Risk factors and risk stratification

Children's Oncology Group Neuroblastoma Risk Stratification is the most commonly used tool to stratify patients based mainly on tumor stage, patient's age, MYCN amplification, DNA index, and tumor histology (**Table 2**) [6].

INSS	INRGSS
Stage 1: localized tumor with complete gross excision; ± microscopic residual disease; representative ipsilateral lymph node negative for tumor microscopically	Stage L1: localized tumor not involving vital structures as defined by IDRFs and confined to one body compartment
Stage 2A: localized tumor with incomplete gross excision; ipsilateral lymph node should be negative for tumor microscopically	Stage L2: locoregional tumor with the presence of one or more IDRFs
Stage 2B: localized tumor with or without complete gross excision; ipsilateral lymph node should be positive for tumor microscopically, while contralateral lymph nodes should be negative microscopically	Equals stage L2
Stage 3: unresectable unilateral tumor crossing the midline, ± involvement of regional lymph node, or localized unilateral tumor with involvement of contralateral regional lymph node or midline tumor with bilateral extension by infiltration (unresectable) or by lymph node involvement	Equals stage L2
Stage 4: primary tumor with dissemination to distant lymph nodes, bone, bone marrow, liver, skin, or other organs	Stage M: distant metastatic disease (except stage MS). Distant lymph node involvement is metastatic disease. Ascites and pleural effusion, even if malignant cells are present, do not constitute metastatic disease unless they are remote from the primary tumor
Stage 4S: localized primary tumor in infants younger than age 1 year (localized as in stage 1, 2A, or 2B) with dissemination limited to the skin, liver, or bone marrow (<10% malignant cells)	Stage MS: metastatic disease in children younger than 547 days (18 months) of age with metastases confined to the skin, liver, and/or bone marrow (<10% malignant cells); MIBG scan must be negative in the bone and bone marrow. Primary tumor can be L1 or L2 with no limitations in terms of crossing or infiltration of the midline

Table 1. Comparison between INSS and INRGSS.

1.3. Multimodal treatment approach for neuroblastoma

1.3.1. Low-risk disease

Low-risk NB patients require minimal therapy; previous pediatric oncology group (POG) and children cancer group (CCG) studies have shown that treatment with surgery alone results in survival rate >95% for patients with stage 1 disease. Even if there is microscopic residual disease, adjuvant treatment with radiotherapy or chemotherapy is not indicated [7, 8]. Diploidy and unfavorable histology predict for local recurrence and, therefore, careful follow-up is necessary, as local recurrence or distant metastasis may rarely occur and require salvage treatment [9].

The primary goals of surgery are to determine an accurate diagnosis, provide accurate surgical staging, completely remove the tumor, offer adjuvant therapy for delayed primary surgery, and remove residual disease with second-look surgery [10].

Management of infrequent patient with stage 1 or 2 with NMYC amplification remains controversial. Although patient with MYCN-amplified stage 1 tumor has significantly event-free survival rate [11], a subset may achieve long-term remission following surgery alone. These rare cases may require continued prospective evaluation to clarify optimal management [12].

1.3.1.1. Stage 4S disease

Infants with stage 4S disease have, in general, a good prognosis; high survival rate has been reported in those infants whose tumor lacks MYCN amplifications [13]. Interestingly Tonini and colleagues reported that, in Italian experience, favorable outcomes were also seen in infants with MYCN-amplified stage 4S neuroblastoma [14]. The tumor may regress spontaneously due to programmed cell death and, therefore treatment is not always necessary. If there are no distressing or life-threatening symptoms, it is possible to follow an observation policy hoping

Stage	Age	MYCN	Ploidy	Histology	Other	Risk group
1						Low
2A/2B		Not amplified			>50% resection	Low
		Not amplified			<50% resection	Intermediate
		Not amplified			Biopsy only	Intermediate
		Amplified				High
3	<547 days	Not amplified				Intermediate
	≥547 days	Not amplified		Favorable		Intermediate
		Amplified				High
	≥547 days	Not amplified		Unfavorable		High
4	<365 days	Amplified				High
	<365 days	Not amplified				Intermediate
	365–547 days	Amplified				High
	365–547 days		DI = 1			High
	365–547 days			Unfavorable		High
	365–547 days	Not amplified	DI > 1	Favorable		Intermediate
	≥547 days					High
4S	<365 days	Not amplified	DI > 1	Favorable	Asymptomatic	Low
	<365 days	Not amplified	DI = 1			Intermediate
	<365 days	Missing	Missing	Missing		Intermediate
	<365 days	Not amplified			Symptomatic	Intermediate
	<365 days	Not amplified		Unfavorable		Intermediate
	<365 days	Amplified				High

Table 2. Children's Oncology Group neuroblastoma risk stratification schema.

for spontaneous regression. Nonintensive chemotherapy is called for if there are major symptoms, e.g., massive hepatomegaly causing respiratory distress. Alternatively, low-dose irradiation may precipitate regression [15].

1.3.1.2. More advanced operable disease

Patients with lymph node involvement, that is, stage 2B and some stage 3 cases, are treated principally by surgery. The need for adjuvant treatment depends on age. In infants <6 months, the role of chemotherapy is controversial. However, in older children, chemotherapy is definitely warranted, using a schedule such as "OPEC," which comprises vincristine, cisplatin, etoposide, and cyclophosphamide [16]. It is often preferable to use chemotherapy as the initial treatment in these patients aiming at reducing the tumor bulk, making complete removal more likely and the surgery safer. Data from POG in patients with stage 2B and stage 3 disease have shown that complete resection is not associated with a significantly better event-free survival than incomplete resection, while patients with favorable Shimada histology have a significantly better event-free survival rate at 2 years than those with unfavorable Shimada (92% versus 58%, respectively) [17].

Irradiation of the tumor bed to eradicate residual disease is controversial.

In a retrospective review of patients with Children's Cancer Study Group (CCSG) stage II disease, no significant benefit was observed in irradiated children [18]. POG designed a randomized trial to evaluate the role of placing radiotherapy in addition to chemotherapy in patients >1 year with nodal disease detected at resection of the primary tumor. Significantly improved local control and survival rates were seen in irradiated children [19]. As the chemotherapy protocol used in this study was less intensive than that now considered standard, it remains possible that more intensive chemotherapy might be as good as combined chemotherapy and radiotherapy in the POG trial. Based on the fact that patients with biologically favorable tumors have a good prognosis [20], even in the presence of residual disease, it is reasonable not to irradiate patients with biologically favorable stage 2B and stage 3 tumors, with or without residual disease after chemotherapy and surgery. Despite the adverse effects of radiotherapy in young children, it should be considered in the treatment plan of patients with biologically unfavorable stage 2B and stage 3 tumors with residual disease [21].

1.3.2. Intermediate-risk disease

Intermediate-risk patients with favorable biology tumors are treated with a short course of chemotherapy (four cycles), while intermediate-risk patients with unfavorable biology receive a longer course of chemotherapy (eight cycles).

In previous POG studies, treatment for infants with regional and metastatic disease was stratified by tumor cell ploidy and MYCN amplification status. Infants with hyperdiploid tumors were treated with cyclophosphamide and doxorubicin, whereas infants with diploid tumors were treated with cisplatin and teniposide after an initial course of cyclophosphamide and doxorubicin [22].

1.3.3. High-risk disease

Survival for high-risk neuroblastoma patients has improved modestly during the past 20 years, although cure rates remain low [23]. This improvement was attributed to intensification of induction chemotherapy, megatherapy consolidation, as well as improved supportive care. Chemotherapy dose intensity has been reported to correlate strongly with both response and progression-free survival where response rates 70–80% have been observed with intensive multiagent induction treatment protocols [24]. Intensification of consolidation therapy with autologous hematopoietic stem cell transplantation following myeloablative conditioning chemotherapy with or without total body irradiation also contributes to improved overall survival in several single-armed studies [25].

Patients with advanced neuroblastoma such as those with stage 4 or inoperable stage 3 disease should receive initial chemotherapy with "OPEC" or a similar protocol. In stage 3 patients, if chemotherapy rendered the tumor operable, it should be removed. In stage 4 patients, surgery to remove residual primary tumor should also be considered complete remission at all metastatic sites has been achieved. Dose intensification treatment strategies, designed to achieve a greater degree of cytoreduction and to circumvent emergence of resistant clones by using a larger number of non-cross-resistant chemotherapeutics in higher doses over a shorter time, are feasible but have not yet proved significantly superior to OPEC [26].

1.3.3.1. Megatherapy

Megatherapy combining high-dose myeloablative chemotherapy and/or total-body irradiation with either autologous bone marrow transplantation or peripheral blood stem cell reinfusion is often used in advanced neuroblastoma. The rationale of megatherapy is to eradicate the undetectable minimal residual disease and prevent disease relapse. Chemotherapeutics at higher-dose levels can bypass inadequate membrane transport and saturate detoxification pathways and DNA repair mechanisms and therefore attack residual tumor cells which have survived initial chemotherapy and became resistant to chemotherapy at conventional doses. Single-agent high-dose melphalan, which was evaluated in European Neuroblastoma Study Group (ENSG) trial 1, is one of the more commonly used conditioning regimens [27].

Radiation, usually in the form of TBI, has been evaluated with high-dose chemotherapy and autologous bone marrow transplantation in treatment of advanced neuroblastoma, and the results were not superior to those achieved by chemotherapy alone, yet the early and late side effects were greater. Allogeneic BMT is not associated with improved results. The European Blood and Marrow Transplant Group has reviewed the data of more than a thousand of neuroblastoma patients who have received myeloablative therapy. Overall, survival was 33% at 5 years, but relapses may still be seen later. When patients relapsed after initial autologous BMT, salvage was not possible, but autologous BMT did salvage 15% of patients in the second or subsequent relapse who had not previously undergone transplantation. The poor outcome for transplantation in stage 4 patients > 1 year is mainly due to persistent skeletal or bone marrow involvement [28].

2. Promising therapeutic targets of neuroblastoma

The 5-year event-free survival for high-risk neuroblastoma is <50%, including children with metastatic neuroblastoma >18 months of age and patients with locoregional or metastatic neuroblastoma with MYCN amplification [5]. Improved outcome was achieved with intensive combination induction chemotherapy and surgery, followed by myeloablative therapy with hematopoietic stem cell transplantation and then differentiation therapy with isotretinoin. Isotretinoin is the first tumor-targeted therapy with established activity in neuroblastoma [29]. After that, a large number of molecular targets have been developed for treatment of high-risk, refractory, and relapsed neuroblastoma. These molecular targets can supplement or replace some of the intensive chemotherapy used for treatment of neuroblastoma.

2.1. Potential advantages of target therapy over conventional chemotherapy

1. Effective cancer treatment with less side effects (increased therapeutic index) due to the targeting of a unique characteristic within the tumor cells, which is usually absent in normal body cells
2. Decreased likelihood of the development of resistance to the targeted therapy due to the molecular target being essential for the viability of the cancer

2.2. Targeting human norepinephrine transporter (hNET) with ^{131}I-metaiodobenzylguanidine (MIBG)

The rationale for using 131 I-MIBG as a targeted radiopharmaceutical for high-risk neuroblastoma was based on the observation that 90% of these tumors are MIBG avid. Studies reported impressive response rates in relapsed disease, and in the largest phase II trial, 37% of patients had a partial response (PR) or complete response (CR) [30].

Many efforts were made to maximize the benefits of MIBG:

a. Increasing tumor radiation dose: the response rate of 42 mCi/kg dose did not appear to be different from that obtained with the standard 18 mCi/kg dose [31].
b. Repeated MIBG infusions: investigators reported a benefit from repeated MIBG infusions given 6–12 weeks apart, with continued improved response in some of the patients with each successive infusion [32].
c. Different isotope (125 I-MIBG): the results were disappointing [33].
d. No carrier added: this approach had the advantage of infusion over 30 min instead of 90–120 min. However, NANT trial showed toxicity, and efficacy profiles equal to those observed with the standard preparation [34].
e. MIBG combined with radiosensitizers or chemotherapy:

- Italian investigators treated 16 children with refractory or relapsed neuroblastoma using ^{131}I-MIBG combined with cisplatin and cyclophosphamide with or without etoposide and vincristine and obtained 12 PRs [35].
- Two studies investigated MIBG combined with a camptothecin, with tolerable toxicity and measurable response [36, 37].
- Combination of a histone deacetylase inhibitor (Vorinostat) with 131I-MIBG showed that Vorinostat at 180 mg/m2/dose is tolerable with 18 mCi/kg MIBG, and A phase II trial comparing this regimen to single-agent MIBG is ongoing [38].
- 131I-MIBG before standard induction therapy with 66% response rate [39].
- 131I-MIBG at the end of induction and before myeloablative therapy for patients with residual MIBG-positive disease reported a response rate of 46% but no improvement in overall survival [40].

2.3. GD2-targeted immunotherapy of high-risk neuroblastoma

Promising results have been emerged with immunotherapy targeting the surface glycolipid molecule disialoganglioside (GD2) that is uniformly expressed by neuroblastomas and gliomas, sarcomas, and some melanomas [41].

GD2 expression is weak in normal human tissues and restricted to neurons, melanocytes, and peripheral pain fibers. Based on this, GD2 seems to be an ideal antigen target for immunotherapy of neuroblastoma [41].

2.3.1. Mechanism of action

a. CDC: complement-dependent cytotoxicity

b. ADCC: antibody-dependent cell cytotoxicity

2.3.1.1. First-generation anti-GD2 mAbs

Many phase I and phase II clinical trials led to the pivotal randomized COG phase III study. This study was conducted on 226 eligible patients to determine whether immunotherapy with ch14.18 combined with GM-CSF, IL-2, and isotretinoin would improve survival compared to isotretinoin alone for children with high-risk neuroblastoma in the first response after myeloablative therapy and stem cell rescue. EFS was significantly higher for patients randomized to immunotherapy, with a 2-year estimated EFS from randomization of 66% versus 46% for patients randomized to isotretinoin alone (P = 0.01). The immunotherapy group also showed significantly higher OS (86% versus 75% at 2 years; P = 0.02). This represents the first successful immunotherapy to target a nonprotein antigen [42].

2.3.1.2. Second-generation anti-GD2 mAbs

Phase II study of Hu14.18-IL-2 immunocytokine showed 5 CRs in 23 neuroblastoma patients evaluable only by bone marrow histology and/or MIBG, but no responses for patients with measurable disease. Preliminary findings of a phase I clinical trial of hu14.18K322 showed reduced neuropathic pain compared to Hu14.18-IL-2 [43].

Yu and colleagues in 2001 carried out a clinical trial of mAb 1A7 as a GD2 vaccine in 31 children with high-risk neuroblastoma who achieved the first or subsequent remissions. No systemic toxicities were observed with subcutaneous injections given periodically over 2 years, and only local reactions were seen. Sixteen of 21 children who enrolled during the first remission had no evidence of disease progression at a median of 6 years, whereas only one of ten children in the second remission remains progression-free. Yu and colleagues concluded that mAb1A7 vaccine is effective at inducing biologically active anti-GD2, has little toxicity, and may be useful for controlling minimal residual disease [44].

2.4. ALK as a therapeutic target in neuroblastoma

Anaplastic lymphoma kinase (ALK) is a tyrosine kinase that is mutated or amplified in about 10% of neuroblastomas and expressed on the surface of most neuroblastoma cells [45].

There are several reasons why inhibition of ALK would be a feasible therapeutic option in neuroblastoma:

1. ALK is expressed on the surface of most neuroblastoma tumor cells and is restricted to the brain following development [45].
2. A proportion of neuroblastoma cells that overexpress phosphorylated ALK that is neither mutated nor amplified respond to ALK depletion by undergoing apoptosis [46].
3. ALK inhibition may provide an effective targeting strategy against MYCN-amplified tumors [47].

Crizotinib was the first drug to be approved by FDA for treatment of ALK-rearranged cancers. Preclinical testing showed the sensitivity of neuroblastoma cell lines with ALK amplification. Crizotinib is being tested in a phase I/II trial for children with neuroblastoma and other solid tumors bearing ALK mutations [48].

2.5. The topoisomerase 1 inhibitors

The topoisomerase 1 inhibitors such as topotecan and irinotecan are often used early for treatment of children with relapsed neuroblastoma because of their acceptable efficacy and toxicity profiles. Topotecan efficacy is enhanced when it is combined with low-dose cyclophosphamide. Irinotecan and temozolomide are a well-tolerated combination, and efficacy is being studied [49].

2.6. Retinoids

A randomized clinical trial of 13-cis-retinoic acid following myeloablative chemotherapy regimen established the importance of retinoids in therapy for high-risk neuroblastoma. Fenretinide produced multi-log cell kill in multiple neuroblastoma cell lines, even those resistant to other retinoids [50]. Phase I studies have shown that fenretinide is generally well tolerated, and COG phase II trial has been completed. Newer formulations of this drug are currently in the pipelines to facilitate oral administration to young children [51].

2.7. Targeting CD133 biomarker

The tumor-initiating properties of CD133 have been discovered through studies such as the one performed by Cournoyer et al. Through genotype analysis CD133 expression is found to be associated with the expression of the Ephrin-A2 (EFNA2) protein. This protein can play a role in cancer development. EFNA2 is expressed in stem cells and can promote the formation of tumors. CD133 and the associated EFNA2 protein are in the pipelines as potential therapeutic targets for neuroblastoma [52].

2.8. Angiogenesis inhibitors

Tumor vascularity has been correlated with aggressiveness in neuroblastoma. Based on this, angiogenesis inhibitors seem to be an attractive therapeutic option. Furthermore, pro-angiogenic molecules appear to be differentially expressed in high-risk tumors, whereas lower-risk tumors are characterized by a stroma that provides anti-angiogenic molecules in the microenvironment. Preclinical studies of anti-angiogenic drugs in neuroblastoma showed promising results [53].

2.9. Targeting insulin-like growth factor I receptor (IGF-IR)

IGF-1R is involved in the regulation of cell proliferation, survival, differentiation, and transformation. IGF-1R is highly expressed in neuroblastoma, and activation of IGF-1R induces MYCN expression. The expression level of IGF-1R has been correlated with tumor metastasis. Blocking IGF-1R with anti-IGF-1R antibodies resulted in the inhibition of neuroblastoma cell growth and tumor regression in neuroblastoma xenograft mouse models. The anti-IGF-1R monoclonal antibody (IMC-A12) is under investigation in phase II trial [54].

2.10. Targeting tropomyosin receptor kinase (TRK)

TRK is now known as the high-affinity receptor for nerve growth factor and as such is crucially involved in the growth, differentiation, and apoptosis of neuronal cells in both the central and the peripheral nervous systems. High expression levels of TRK have been correlated with poor outcome in neuroblastoma and chemotherapy resistance. Several TRK-blocking small compounds, such as CEP-701, have been developed. Blocking TRK using CEP-701 results in induction of apoptosis and growth inhibition of human neuroblastoma xenografts in nude mice. CEP-701 is under investigation in phase I trial for refractory and relapsed neuroblastoma. Other tyrosine kinase inhibitors, including inhibitors of the epidermal growth factor receptor, might have activity against neuroblastoma [55]. Imantanib mesylate has also been investigated in neuroblastoma because some tumors appear to express c-kit, PDGFR, or both; however, activating mutations in these receptors have not been reported [56].

2.11. Targeting Aurora A kinase (AURKA)

AURKA is a serine/threonine kinase, which stabilizes the microtubule at the spindle pole during segregation of chromosomes. Based on this, AURKA is essential for G2-M progression, and its inhibition results in cell cycle arrest and apoptosis. AURKA is overexpressed in neuroblastoma, and amplification of its gene has also been observed in neuroblastoma cells. In phase I trials, promising results have also been obtained with AURKA inhibitor MLN8237 [57].

2.12. Targeting PI3K/AKT/mTOR pathway

The PI3K/AKT/mTOR pathway is an intracellular signaling pathway important in regulating the cell cycle. Therefore, it is directly related to cellular quiescence, proliferation, cancer, and longevity. PI3K activation phosphorylates and activates AKT that sequentially activates mTOR. In many cancers, this pathway is overactive, thus reducing apoptosis and allowing proliferation. Rapamycin (Sirolimus), an antifungal agent with immunosuppressive properties, was first isolated in 1975 from the soil of the island of Rapa Nui or Easter Island. In the 1980s, rapamycin showed a broad anticancer activity. However, clinical development of rapamycin as an anticancer agent was hampered by unfavorable pharmacokinetics. Recent development of rapamycin analogs with favorable pharmacokinetics such as temsirolimus, everolimus, and ridaforolimus opened up the present era of mTOR inhibitors as anticancer agents [58].

2.13. Other strategies

Epigenetic silencing of genes that are crucial for induction of apoptosis, such as caspase-8, seems to occur frequently in neuroblastoma. Therefore, demethylating agents such as decitabine are currently being investigated. Histone deacetylase inhibitors showed preclinical activity against neuroblastoma. More than three histone deacetylase inhibitors are now in clinical trials for patients with refractory solid tumors. Heat shock protein 90 inhibitors are also of interest because they alter the function of molecules associated with neuroblastoma cell growth and proliferation, including AKT, IGF-1, and TrkB [59].

Author details

Tamer Hassan*, Mohamed Badr, Usama El Safy, Mervat Hesham, Laila Sherief, Mohamed Beshir, Manar Fathy, Mohamed Al Malky and Marwa Zakaria

*Address all correspondence to: dr.tamerhassan@yahoo.com

Department of Pediatrics, Zagazig University, Egypt

References

[1] Gumus K. A child with raccoon eyes masquerading as trauma. International Ophthalmology. 2007;**27**:379-381

[2] Heck JE, Ritz B, Hung RJ, Hashibe M, Boffetta P. The epidemiology of neuroblastoma: A review. Paediatric and Perinatal Epidemiology. 2009;**23**(2):125-143

[3] Gains J, Mandeville H, Cork N, Brock P, Gaze M. Ten challenges in the management of neuroblastoma. Future Oncology. 2012;**8**(7):839-858

[4] Brodeur GM, Pritchard J, Berthold F, Carlsen NL, Castel V, Castelbenv RP, De Bernard B, Evans AE, Favrot M, Hedborg F, et al. Revisions of the international criteria for neuroblastoma diagnosis, staging, and response to treatment. Progress in Clinical and Biological Research. 1994;**385**:363-369

[5] Cohn SL, Pearson AD, London WB, Monclair T, Ambros PF, Brodeur GM, Faldum A, Hero B, Iehara T, Machin D, Mosseri V, Simon T, Garaventa A, Castel V, Matthay KK; INRG Task Force. The International Neuroblastoma Risk Group (INRG) classification system: An INRG Task Force report. Journal of Clinical Oncology. 2009;**27**(2):289-297

[6] London WB, Castleberry RP, Matthay KK, Look AT, Seeger RC, Shimada H, Thomer P, Brodeur G, Maris JM, Reynolds CP, Cohn SL. Evidence for an age cutoff greater than 365 days for neuroblastoma risk group stratification in the Children's Oncology Group. Journal of Clinical Oncology. 2005;**23**(27):6459-6465

[7] Ninane J, Pritchard J, Morris Jones PH, Mann JR, Malpas JS. Stage 11 neuroblastoma: Adverse prognostic significance of lymph node involvement. Archives of Disease in Childhood. 1982;**57**(6):438-442

[8] Haves FA, Green A, Hustu HO, Kumar M. Surgicopathologic staging of neuroblastoma: Prognostic significance of regional lymph node metastases. Journal of Pediatrics. 1983;**102**(1):59-62

[9] Cheung NK, Kushner BH, LaQuaglia MP, Kramer K, Ambros P, Ambros I, Ladanyi M, Eddv J, Bonilla MA, Gerald W. Survival from non-stage 4 neuroblastoma without cytotoxic therapy: An analysis of clinical and biological markers. European Journal of Cancer. 1997;**33**(12):2117-2120

[10] Nitschke R, Smith EI, Shochat S, Altshuler G, Travers H, Shuster JJ, Haves FA, Pattcrson R, McWilliams N. Localized neuroblastoma treated by surgery: A Pediatric Oncology Group Study. Journal of Clinical Oncology. 1988;**6**(8):1271-1279

[11] Alvarado CS, London WB, Look AT, Brodew GM, Altmiller DH, Thomer PS, Joshi VV, Rowe ST, Nash MB, Smith EL, Castleberrv RP, Cohn SL. Natural history and biology of stage A neuroblastoma: A Pediatric Oncology Group study. Journal of Pediatric Hematology/Oncology. 2000;**22**(3):197-205

[12] Perez CA, Matthay KK, Atkinson JB, Seeger RC, Shimada H, Haase GM, Stram DO, Gerbing RB, Lukens JN. Biologic variables in the outcome of stages I and II neuroblastoma treated with surgery as primary therapy: A Children's Cancer Group study. Journal of Clinical Oncology. 2000;**18**(1):18-26

[13] Nickerson HJ, Matthay KK, Seeger RC, Brodeur GM, Shimada H, Perez Q, Atkinson JB, Selch M, Gerbing RB, Stram DO, Lukens J. Favorable biology and outcome of stage IV-S neuroblastoma with supportive care or minimal therapy: A Children's Cancer Group study. Journal of Clinical Oncology. 2000;**18**(3):477-486

[14] Tonini GP, Boni L, Pession A, Rogers D, Iolascon A, Basso G, Cordero di Montezemolo L, Casale F, Pession A, Perri P, Mazzocco K, Scaruffi P, Lo Cunsolo C, Marchese N, Milanaccio C, Conte M, Bruzzi P, De Bemardi B. MYCN oncogene amplification in neuroblastoma is associated with worse prognosis, except in stage 4s: The Italian experience with 295 children. Journal of Clinical Oncology. 1997;**15**(1):85-93

[15] Yamamoto K, Hanada R, Kikuchi A, Ichikawa M, Aihara T, Oguma E, Moritani T, Shimanuki Y, Tanimura M, Havashi Y. Spontaneous regression of localized neuroblastoma detected by mass screening. Journal of Clinical Oncology. 1998;**16**(4):1265-1269

[16] Shafford EA, Rogers OW, Pritchard J. Advanced neuroblastoma: Improved response rate using a multiagent regimen (OPEC) including sequential cisplatin and VM-26. Journal of Clinical Oncology. 1984;**2**(7):742-747

[17] Strother D, van Hoff J, Rao PV, Smith EI, Shamberger RC, Halperin EC, Murray KJ, Castleberry RP. Event-free survival of children with biologically favourable neuroblastoma based on the degree of initial tumor resection: Results from the Pediatric Oncology Group. European Journal of Cancer. 1997;**33**(12):2121-2125

[18] Matthay KK, Sather HN, Seeger RC, Haase GM, Hammond GD. Excellent outcome of stage II neuroblastoma is independent of residual disease and radiation therapy. Journal of Clinical Oncology. 1989;**7**(2):236-244

[19] Castlebeny RP, Kun LE, Schuster JJ, Altshuler G, Smith LE, Nitschke R, Wharam M, McWilliams N, Joshi V, Hayes FA. Radiotherapy improves the outlook for patients older than 1 year with Pediatric Oncology Group Stage C neuroblastoma. Journal of Clinical Oncology. 1991;**9**(5):789-795

[20] Strother O, van Hoff J, Rao PV, Smith ET, Shamberger RC, Halperin EC, Murray KJ, Castleberry RP. Event-free survival of children with biologically favourable neuroblastoma based on the degree of initial tumor resection: Results from the Pediatric Oncology Group. European Journal of Cancer. 1997;**33**(12):2121-2125

[21] Matthay KK, Perez C, Seeger RC, Brodeur GM, Shimada H, Atkinson JB, Black CT, Gerbing R, Haase GM, Stram DO, Swift P, Lukens JN. Successful treatment of Stage III neuroblastoma based on prospective biological staging: A Children's Cancer Group study. Journal of Clinical Oncology. 1998;**16**(4):1256- 1264

[22] Bowman LC, Castleberry RP, Cantor A, Joshi V, Cohn SL, Smith EI, Yu A, Brodeur GM, Hayes FA, Look AT. Genetic staging of unresectable or metastatic neuroblastoma in infants: A Pediatric Oncology Group study. Journal of the National Cancer Institute. 1997;**89**(5):373-380

[23] Frappaz D, Michon J, Coze C, Berger C, Plouvier E, Lasset C, Bemard JL, Stephan JL, Bouffet E, Buclon M, Combaret V, Fourquet A, Philip L Zucker JM. LMCE3 treatment strategy: Results in 99 consecutively diagnosed stage 4 neuroblastomas in children older than 1 year at diagnosis. Journal of Clinical Oncology. 2000;**18**(3):468-476

[24] Kushner BH, LaQuaglia MP, Bonilla MA, Lindslev K, Rosenfield N, Yeh S, Eddv J, Gerald WL, Heller G, Cheung NK. Highly effective induction therapy for stage 4 neuroblastoma in children over I year of age. Journal of Clinical Oncology. 1994;**12**(12):2607-2613

[25] Ladenstein R, Philip T, Lasset C, Hartmann O, Garaventa A, Pinkerton R, Michon J, Pritchard J, Klingebiel T, Kremens B, Pearson A, Coze C, Paolucci P, Frappaz D, Gadner H, Chauvin F, et al. Multivariate analysis of risk factors in stage 4 neuroblastoma patients over the age of one year treated with megatherapy and stem-cell transplantation: A report from the European Bone Marrow Transplantation Solid Tumor Registry. Journal of Clinical Oncology. 1998;**16**(3):953-965

[26] Pinkerton CR, Zucker JM, Hartmann O, Pritchard J, Broadbent V, Morris-Jones P, Breatnach F, Craft AE, Pearson AD, Wallendszus KR, et al. Short duration, high dose, alternating chemotherapy in metastatic neuroblastoma. (ENSG 3C induction regimen). The European neuroblastoma study group. British Journal of Cancer. 1990;**62**(2):319-323

[27] Pritchard J, Cotterill SJ, Germond SM, Imeson J, de Kraker J, Jones DR. High dose melphalan in the treatment of advanced neuroblastoma: Results of a randomized trial (ENSG- 1) by the European Neuroblastoma Study Group. Pediatric Blood & Cancer. 2005;**44**(4):348-357

[28] Philip T, Ladenstein R, Lasset C, Hartmann O, Zucker JM, Pinkerton R, Pearson AD, Klingebiel T, Garaventa A, Kremens B, Bernard JL, Rosti G, Chauvin F. 1070 myeloablative megatherapy procedures followed by stem cell rescue for neuroblastoma: 17 years of European experience and conclusions. European Journal of Cancer. 1997;**33**(12):2130-2135

[29] Matthay KK, Villablanca JG, Seeger RC, Stram DO, Han-is RE, Ramsay NK, Swift P, Shimada H, Black CT, Brodeur OM, Gerbing RB, Reynolds CP. Treatment of high-risk neuroblastoma with intensive chemotherapy, radiotherapy, autologous bone marrow transplantation, and 13-cis-retinoic acid. Children's Cancer Group. The New England Journal of Medicine. 1999;**341**(16):1165-1173

[30] Matthay KK, Shulkin B, Ladcnstcin R, Michon J, Giammarilc E, Lewington V, Pearson AD, Cohn SL. Criteria for evaluation of disease extent by (123)I-metaiodobenzylguanidine scans in neuroblastoma: A report for the International Neuroblastoma Risk Group (INRG) Task Force. British Journal of Cancer. 2010;**102**(9):1319-1326

[31] Matthay KK, Quach A, Huberty J, Franc BL, Hawkins RA, Jackson H, Groshen S, Shustennan S, Yanik G, Veatch J, Brophv P, Yillablanca JG, Maris JM. Iodine-131-

metaiodobenzylguanidine double infusion with autologous stem-cell rescue for neuroblastoma: A new approach to neuroblastoma therapy phase I study. Journal of Clinical Oncology. 2009;**27**(7):1020-1025

[32] Howard JP, Maris JM, Kersun LS, Hubertv JP, Cheng SC, Hawkins RA, Matthay KK. Tumor response and toxicity with multiple infusions of high dose (131) I-MIBG for refractory neuroblastoma. Pediatric Blood & Cancer. 2005;**44**(3):232-239

[33] Sisson JC, Shapiro B, Hutchinson RJ, Zasadny KR, Mallette S, Mudgett EE, Wieland DM. Treatment of neuroblastoma with [^{125}I] metaiodobenzylguanidine. The Journal of Nuclear Biology and Medicine. 1991;**35**(4):255-259

[34] Matthay KK, Weiss B, Maris J, Maris JM, Yanik GA, Dubois SO, Stubbs J, Groshen S, Tsao-Wei D, Hawkins R, Jackson H, Goodarzian F, Daldrup-Link H, Panigrahy A, Towbin A, Shimada H, Barrett J, Lafrance N, Babich J. Dose escalation study of no-carrier added 131 I Metaiodobenzylguanidine (131 I-MIBG) for relapsed or refractory neuroblastoma: A New Approaches to Neuroblastoma Therapy (NANT)Trial. Journal of Nuclear Medicine. 2012;**53**(7):1155-1163

[35] Mastrangelo S, Tomesello A, Diociaiuti L, Pession A, Prete A, Rufini V, Troncone L, Mastrangelo R. Treatment of advanced neuroblastoma: Feasibility and therapeutic potential of a novel approach combining 131 1-MIBG and multiple drug chemotherapy. British Journal of Cancer. 2001;**84**(4):460-464

[36] Gaze MN, Chang YC, Flux GD, Mairs RJ, Saran FH, Meller ST. Feasibility of dosimetry-based high-dose 131 I-metaiodobenzylguanidine with topotecan as a radiosensitizer in children with metastatic neuroblastoma. Cancer Biotherapy and Radiopharmaceuticals. 2005;**20**(2):195-199

[37] Dubois SG, Chesler L, Groshen S, Hawkins R, Goodarzian F, Shimada H, Yanik G, Tallen M, Stewart C, Mosse YP, Maris JM, Tsao-Wei D, Marachelian A, Villablanca JG, Matthav KK. Phase I study of vincristine, irinotecan, and 131 I-metaiodobenzylguanidine (131 I-MIBG) for patients with relapsed or refractory neuroblastoma: A New Approaches to Neuroblastoma Therapy (NANT) trial. Clinical Cancer Research. 2012;**18**(9):2679-2686

[38] Bhargava S, Mueller S, Wehmeijer L, Yang X, Gragg A, Matthay KK, Weiss WA, Haas-Kogan DA. PARP-1 inhibitor MK-4827 in combination with radiation is a novel treatment strategy of metastatic neuroblastoma. Journal of Clinical Oncology. 2011:**29** (suppl; abstr 9559)

[39] de Kraker T, Hoefnagel KA, Verschuur AC, van Eck B, van Santen HM, Caron HN. Iodine-131 metaiodobenzylguanidine as initial induction therapy in stage 4 neuroblastoma patients over 1 year of age. European Journal of Cancer. 2008;**44**(4):551-556

[40] Schmidt M, Simon T, Hero B, Eschner W, Dietlein M, Sudbrock F, Bongartz R, Betthold F, Schicha H. Is there a benefit of 131 I-MIBG therapy in the treatment of children with stage 4 neuroblastoma? A retrospective evaluation of the German Neuroblastoma Trial NB97 and implications for the German Neuroblastoma Trial NB2004. Nuklearmedizin. 2006;**45**(4):145-151

[41] Svennerholm L, Bostrom K, Fredman P, Jungbjer B, Lekman A, Månsson JE, Rynmark BM. Gangliosides and allied glycosphingolipids in human peripheral nerve and spinal cord. Biochimica et Biophysica Acta. 1994;**1214**(2):115-123

[42] Yu AL, Gilman AL, Ozkavnak MF, London WB, Kreissman SG, Chen HX, Smith M, Anderson B, Villablanca JG, Matthay KK, Shimada H, Grupp SA, Seeger R, Revnolds CP, Buxton A, Reisfeld RA, Gillies SD, Cohn SL, Maris JM, Sondel PM; Children's Oncologv Group. Anti-GD2 antibody with GM-CSF, interleukin-2, and isotretinoin for neuroblastoma. The New England Journal of Medicine. 2010;**363**(14):1324-1334

[43] Shusterman S, London WB, Gillies SD, Hank JA, Voss SD, Seeger RC, Reynolds CP, Kimball J, Albeltini MR, Wagner B, Gan J, Eickhoff J, De Santes KB, Cohn SL, Hecht T, Gadbaw B, Reisfeld RA, Maris JM, Sondel PM. Antitumor activity of hu14.l8-IL2 in patients with relapsed/refractory neuroblastoma: Children's Oncology Group (COG) phase II study. Journal of Clinical Oncology. 2010;**28**(33):4969-4975

[44] Yu AL, Eskenazi A, Strother D, Castleberry R. A pilot study of anti idiotype monoclonal anti body as tumor vaccine in patients with high risk neuroblastoma. Proceeding of American Society of Clinical Oncology. 2001;**20**:(abstract 1470)

[45] Lamant L, Pulford K, Bischo FD, Morris SW, Mason DY, Delsol G, Mariame B. Expression of the ALK tyrosine kinase gene in neuroblastoma. The American Journal of Pathology. 2000;**156**(5):1711-1721

[46] Passoni L, Longo L, Collini P, Coluccia AM, Bozzi F, Podda M, Gregorio A, Gambini C, Garaventa A, Pistoia V, Del Grosso F, Tonini GB, Cheng M, Gambacorti-Passerini C, Anichini A, Fossati-Bellan IF, Di Nicola M, Luksch R. Mutation-independent anaplastic lymphoma kinase overexpression in poor prognosis neuroblastoma patients. Cancer Research. 2009;**69**(18):7338-7346

[47] De Brouwer S, De Preter K, Kumps C, Zabrocki P, Porcu M, Westerhout EM, et al. Meta-analysis of neuroblastomas reveals a skewed ALK mutation spectrum in tumors with MYCN amplification. Clinical Cancer Research. 2010;**16**(17):4353-4362

[48] Bresler SC, Wood AC, Haglund EA, Courtright J, Belcastro LT, Plegaria JS, et al. Differential inhibitor sensitivity of anaplastic lymphoma kinase variants found in neuroblastoma. Science Translational Medicine. 2011;**3**(108):108-114

[49] Langler A, Christaras A, Abshagen K, Krauth K, Hero B, Berthold F. Topotecan in the treatment of refractory neuroblastoma and other malignant tumors in childhood—A phase-IT-study. Klinische Pädiatrie. 2002;**214**(4):153-156

[50] Reynolds CP, Matthay KK, Villablanca JG, Maurer BJ. Retinoid therapy of high-risk neuroblastoma. Cancer Letters. 2003;**197**(l-2):185-192

[51] Garaventa AL, Luksch R, Lo Piccolo MS, Cavadini E, Montaldo PG, Pizzitola MR, Boni L, Ponzoni M, Decensi A, De Bernard IB, Bellani FF, Formelli F. Phase I trial and pharmacokinetics of fenretinide in children with neuroblastoma. Clinical Cancer Research. 2001;**9**(6):2012-2019

[52] Cournoyer S, Nyalendo C, Addioui A, Belounis A, Beaunover M, Aumont A, Teira P, Duval M, Fernandes K, Fetni R, Haddad E, Sallelet H. Genotype analysis of tumor-initiating cells expressing CD 133 in neuroblastoma. Genes, Chromosomes & Cancer. 2012;**51**(8):792-804

[53] Chlenski A, Liu S, Crawford SE, Volpert OV, DeVries GH, Evangelista A, Yang Q, Salwen HR, Farrer R, Bray J, Cohn SL. SPARC is a key Schwannian-derived inhibitor controlling neuroblastoma tumor angiogenesis. Cancer Research. 2002;**62**(24):7357-7363

[54] Geoerger B, Brasme JF, Daudigeos-Dubus E, Opolon P, Venot C, Debussche L, Vrignaud P, Vassal G. Anti-insulin-like growth factor l receptor antibody EM 164 (murine AVE1642) exhibits anti-tumor activity alone and in combination with temozolomide against neuroblastoma . European Journal of Cancer. 2010;**46**(18):3251-3262

[55] Ho R, Minturn JE, Hishiki T, Zhao H, Wang Q, Cnaan A, Maris J, Evans AE, Brodeur GM. Proliferation of human neuroblastomas mediated by the epidermal growth factor receptor. Cancer Research. 2005;**65**(21):9868-9875

[56] Beppu K, Jaboine J, Merchant MS, Mackall CL, Thiele CJ. Effect of imatinib mesylate on neuroblastoma tumorigenesis and vascular endothelial growth factor expression. Journal of the National Cancer Institute. 2004;**96**(1):46-55

[57] Carol H, Boehm I, Revnolds CP, Kang MH, Maris JM, Morton CL, Gorlick R, Kolb EA, Keir ST, Wu J Wozniak AE, Yang Y, Manfredi M, Ecsedy J, Wang J, Neale G, Houghton PJ, Smith MA, Lock RB. Efficacy and pharmacokinetic/pharmacodynamic evaluation of the Aurora kinase A inhibitor MLN8237 against preclinical models of pediatric cancer. Cancer Chemotherapy and Pharmacology. 2011;**68**(5):1291-1304

[58] Porta C, Paglino C, Mosca A. Targeting PI3K/Akt/mTOR signaling in cancer. Frontiers in Oncology. 2014;**14**(4):64

[59] Bagatell R, Beliakoff J, David CL, Marron MT, Whitesell L. Hsp90 inhibitors deplete key anti-apoptotic proteins in pediatric solid tumor cells and demonstrate synergistic anticancer activity with cisplatin. International Journal of Cancer. 2005;**113**(2):179-188

Chapter 5

Molecular Approach to Neuroblastoma

Bakiye Goker Bagca and Cigir Biray Avci

Additional information is available at the end of the chapter

http://dx.doi.org/10.5772/intechopen.69374

Abstract

Neuroblastoma is a notably malignant cancer originates from neuroblastoma stem cells during embryogenesis. It can originate from any region of the peripheral nervous system. Neuroblastoma is a heterogeneous cancer. The cells responsible for heterogeneous structure are neuroblastoma stem cells that initiate the cancer and generate into all the cancer cells and have self-renewal property. Although some specific surface markers and genetic patterns of neuroblastoma stem cell were determined, all mechanisms have not been illuminated yet. Mutations that are specific to neuroblastoma development, risk group, and disease-stage are identified. However, epigenetic dysregulations also play major roles in the development of neuroblastoma. Patients gradually develop resistance to conventional chemotherapy or relapse occurs after treatment. New therapy approaches have been developed, either as alternatives to conventional chemotherapy, or in combination with it, in order to overcome the handicaps. Targeted therapies, those directly affecting the cancer cell or the cancer stem cell and having a minimal effect on healthy cells, constitute these approaches. Since neuroblastoma is highly heterogeneous both genetically and epigenetically, the data obtained from molecular mechanisms will greatly contribute to the survival of patients.

Keywords: neuroblastoma, neuroblastoma stem cell, molecular, epigenetic, miRNA, lncRNA, targeted therapy

1. Introduction

Neuroblastoma is a type of neural crest originated cancer, can arise in any region of the sympathetic nervous system, but occurs in more than 50% of adrenal glands. Metastasis usually occurs to the lymph nodes, bone marrow, bones and rarely to the lung, liver, and central nervous system. Metastasis is the most important factor that decreases survival rates to 40%. Clinical symptoms can vary according to the primary tumor site and the site of metastasis.

INTECH
open science | open minds

© 2017 The Author(s). Licensee InTech. This chapter is distributed under the terms of the Creative Commons Attribution License (http://creativecommons.org/licenses/by/3.0), which permits unrestricted use, distribution, and reproduction in any medium, provided the original work is properly cited. (cc) BY

Incidence and phenotype of the disease vary by the age, sex, and ethnicities; however, neuroblastoma is regarded as an orphan disease, with approximately eight cases per million in the worldwide and these cases comprise 7% of all childhood cancers. The maximal rate of the cases occurs in the perinatal age. The median age of the neuroblastoma is 18 months and 90% of the patients are under 10 years of age. When seen in adolescents who constitute 5% of all cases, usually exhibit chemotherapy-resistant character.

With the International Neuroblastoma Pathology Committee (INPC) modification of the Shimada classification of 1984, the neuroblastoma was divided into four categories according to morphological and biological characteristics of the cells, and patient age: neuroblastoma, intermixed ganglioneuroblastoma, ganglioneuroma, and nodular ganglioneuroblastoma. Although many different staging systems have been used in the past, International Neuroblastoma Staging System (INSS), including 1, 2A, 2B, 3, 4 and 4S stages, which are formed according to tumor size and metastasis status, is currently used. By combining the disease stages with prognostic factors, very low, low, medium, high-risk groups were formed.

The spontaneous regression has been observed for patients with stage 4S who have limited metastatic characteristics below 1 year of age. Neuroblastoma is less common but more malignant in people with African ancestry than European ones. Moreover, the disease is infrequent in girls than in boys. However, genetic, epigenetic, and environmental factors, which affect the incidence, have not been openly described yet.

Although neuroblastoma is initially considered a familial disease, it is now known that familial cases constitute only 1% of all cases. In particular, germline gain-of-function mutations of the anaplastic lymphoma receptor tyrosine kinase (ALK) and paired like homeobox 2b (PHOX2B) genes are responsible for these familial events, while neuroblastoma has been described as a complex disease resulting from combination of many different allelic effects.

Neuroblastoma is originated from the neuroblastoma stem cell, which is the resultant genetic alterations of progenitor cells that will differentiate into the sympathetic nervous system. The amplification of the V-Myc Avian Myelocytomatosis Viral Oncogene Neuroblastoma-Derived Homolog (MYCN) gene, a transcriptional regulator that promotes cell cycle and differentiation, induces activation of oncogenes and inhibition of tumor suppressors, is the most common genetic alteration in neuroblastoma. MYCN amplification has been associated with tumor grade, progression, and metastasis. ALK mutations also play a role in neuroblastoma pathology, leading to the activation of oncogenic signaling pathways by somatic amplification as well as familial predisposition. Polymorphisms and overexpression of the Lin-28 Homolog B (LIN28B) gene, involved in the regulation of multiple signaling pathways, play a role in neuroblastoma formation and progression more often than amplification. Loss-of-function mutations in the transcriptional regulator Chromatin Remodeler (ATRX) gene, regulation in the promoter region of the telomerase enzyme Telomerase Reverse Transcriptase (TERT) gene, mutations in genes involved in chromatin remodeling are associated with neuroblastoma development and progression. Somatic mutations in noncoding regions as much as in coding regions have also been associated with neuroblastoma progression. In particular, mutations in noncoding regions of tumor suppressor and candidate tumor suppressor genes are highly effective on high-risk neuroblastoma.

Laboratory tests, radiographic imaging, and histological staining methods are used in the diagnosis of neuroblastoma, staging, and monitoring the treatment. The increased levels of catecholamine and its metabolites in urine are the most commonly used biomarkers in neuroblastoma. More rarely, increased levels of adrenaline derivatives are found in the plasma. Radiological approaches as ultrasonography, CT, and MRI are used for staging and metastatic profiling. Molecular analysis of genes such as MYCN, ALK is also important in diagnosis and routine monitoring. For this purpose, mutations in biopsy specimens can be detected at single cell level using Fluorescence In Situ Hybridization (FISH), real-time Polymerase Chain Reaction (PCR), flow cytometry, Single-nucleotide polymorphism (SNP) arrays, Next-Generation Sequencing (NGS), and microarray methods.

Neuroblastoma treatment includes surgical removal of the primer tumor, standard chemotherapy, and induction chemotherapy, autologous hematopoietic stem cell transplantation following by myeloablative chemotherapy and radiotherapy approaches, depending on the risk group of the patients. Unfortunately, over time, resistance to chemotherapeutics occurs in the patient and relapses frequently occur after the treatment. To overcome these handicaps, research for neuroblastoma treatment has been focused on targeted therapy strategies to improve survival of patients.

2. Molecular pathology of neuroblastoma

The most common genetic and epigenetic alterations in neuroblastoma include MYCN, ALK, PHOX2B, ATRX, TERT, Tumor Protein P53 (TP53), Lysine methyltransferases (KMTs), Histone lysine demethylases (KDMs), and Histone deacetylase (HDAC) genes, noncoding RNA (ncRNA) expression changes [1]. Although only a few mutations that define neuroblastoma development, prognosis, and metastatic characteristics have been identified, many of the genetic alterations underlying this rare disease remain to be discovered yet to improve treatment success and patient survival. With the development of novel methods in the molecular medicine in recent years, the studies in this area and the resulting findings are rapidly increasing and allow for the development of promising approaches in the treatment.

2.1. Neuroblastoma-specific genetic alterations

Amplification of the MYCN proto-oncogene has been the first discovered aberration associated with neuroblastoma pathogenesis. In a study realized by Brodeur et al. in 1984, it was determined that the DNA copy number of the MYCN gene in the human neuroblastoma cell line is 20–140 times amplified, unlike other human cancer cell lines. In accordance with the result, they showed that the copy number of MYCN is correlated with the disease stage and poor prognosis in untreated patients [2].

The MYCN proto-oncogene, also referred to as N-myc, localized in 2p24.3, is a transcription factor that is homologous to the MYC (c-MYC) proto-oncogene localized in 8q24.21, whose mutations have been associated with hematological malignancies and lymphomas [3, 4]. MYCN alterations have been related with various solid tumors, especially neuroblastoma. It is localized in the nucleus and activates transcription of many genes that support cell survival and proliferation via dimerization with the other transcription factors, which have the same binding domain. It also suppresses the genes responsible for normal cell differentiation [5]. Accumulation of neuroblasts with the impairment of normal differentiation of neuronal cells is the underlying cause of primer neuroblastoma formation.

Familial neuroblastomas rarely occur and constitute approximately 1–2% of all cases. The tyrosine kinase receptor ALK, which plays an essential role in the development of the normal brain and nervous system, is the major component of hereditary neuroblastomas [6]. However, abnormal ALK expression plays an important role not only in hereditary neuroblastoma but also in the development of sporadic neuroblastoma [7].

In addition to ALK, PHOX2B gene, the main regulator of neural crest development is responsible for the development of familial neuroblastoma [8].

While MYCN amplification is responsible for a large proportion of sporadic neuroblastomas (~20%), a large proportion of adolescent and young adult patients have ATRX mutations (~20%) without MYCN amplification [9]. ATRX, a chromatin remodeling gene that is a member of the SWI/SNF family, plays a role in the regulation of gene expression by the epigenetic mechanism by organizing the matrix-chromatin interaction [10]. ATRX is responsible for H3.3 accumulation in methylation silencing regions such as transposon elements, imprinted genes, and telomeres [11]. Telomere-repeat sequences are located at the end regions of the chromosomes and maintain the stability of the chromosomes. In eukaryotic cells, telomeres are shortened at each replication, thus limiting the proliferation ability of the cell [12]. There are two mechanisms involved in maintaining the telomere length, which leads to the proliferation capacity of both stem/progenitor cells and cancer cells.

First, these are the activation of the alternative lengthening of telomeres (ALT) mechanism, which involves the loss of function of the ATRX gene. Mutations of the ATRX gene cause abnormally long telomere lengths in cancers, including neuroblastoma [13].

The second mechanism that plays a role in the conservation of telomere length is the activation of the telomerase enzyme by rearrangement of the TERT gene. Mutations in the TERT gene are highly associated with high-stage neuroblastoma patients (~20%) who do not have MYCN and ATRX mutations and are associated with poor prognosis [14].

The catastrophic process, called chromothripsis, describes a new carcinogenesis mechanism that is caused by a large number (tens to hundreds) of rearrangements occurring in the same cell in one or several chromosomes, unlike the conventional mechanism in which the accumulation of mutations over time causes cancer [15]. Chromothripsis mechanisms have been highly defined through recent whole-genome sequencing studies. Defects that play a role in the mechanism occur in genes that are involved in nervous system development and neuritogenesis. Defects of the transmembrane protein tyrosine phosphatase, receptor type D (PTPRD), teneurin transmembrane protein 2 (TENM2), teneurin transmembrane protein 3 (TENM3), CUB and sushi multiple domains 1 (CSMD1) proteins which play a role in nervous system development and T-cell lymphoma invasion and metastasis 1 (TIAM1), Rho GTPase activating protein (DLC1) GTPase proteins involved in Rac/Rho signaling through these transmembrane proteins are responsible for the development of high-grade neuroblastoma without MYCN amplification. Down regulation of the cell division cycle 42 (CDC42) gene, a GTPase located in 1p36, is characterized in advanced disease patients with MYCN amplification [16].

In addition to CDC42, 1p36 deletion including RhoGEF kinase (KALRN), calmodulin binding transcription activator 1 (CAMTA1), kinesin family member 1B (KIF1B), castor zinc finger 1 (CASZ1) genes and 17q acquisition are correlated with MYCN amplification in the high-stage neuroblastoma [17, 18]. 11q loss of heterozygosity that is inversely related to MYCN amplification is also responsible for a large proportion of high-stage neuroblastoma.

Large spectrum of genetic-wide association studies has identified many genetic alterations related to predisposition to nonfamilial (sporadic) neuroblastomas, recently. The genes associated with genetic predisposition are BRCA1-associated RING domain 1 (BARD1), which regulates tumor suppressor BRCA1 activity, transcriptional regulator LIM domain only 1 (LMO1), dual specificity phosphatase 12 (DUSP12) that controls cell proliferation, DEAD-box helicase 4 (DDX4), a helicase that regulates the secondary structure of RNA and its associated functions, interleukin 31 receptor A (IL31RA), hydroxysteroid 17-beta dehydrogenase 12 (HSD17B12) which plays role in fatty acid biosynthesis, HECT Domain and ankyrin repeat containing E3 ubiquitin protein ligase 1 (HACE1) that regulates proteosomal degredation, LIN28B, neurofilament light (NEFL) that plays a role in the formation of neurons and TP53 gene, one of the most important transcription factor and a tumor suppressor that regulates essential cellular events as apoptosis, DNA repair [19–21].

2.2. Epigenetic pattern in neuroblastoma

Epigenetic modifications are reversible changes that play a role in the regulation of gene expression by regulating the chromatin accessibility of the elements necessary for transcription in eukaryotic cells via chromatin remodeling, histone modifications, DNA methylation, and noncoding RNAs. While acetylation is only associated with euchromatin, methylation regulates both euchromatin and heterochromatin [22].

Results from microarray-based DNA methylation studies performed in neuroblastoma patients have shown that gene-specific (promoter) hypomethylation occurs more frequently than genomic hypermethylation that cause development of neuroblastoma [23, 24]. Both upregulation and downregulation of the DNA methyltransferases may be associated with the pathogenesis of neuroblastoma, depending on the functions of the genes which have promoter methylation. O-6-methylguanine-DNA methyltransferase (MGMT), a DNA methyltransferase, interacting with the Wnt/B-catenin signaling pathway is upregulated in the neuroblastoma and is associated with chemotherapy resistance [25]. However, DNA methyltransferase 3 beta (DNMT3B7), a DNA methyltransferase, regulates genomic methylation in neuroblastoma and triggers normal neuronal differentiation [26].

Similar to DNA methylation, histone methylation and demethylation have different effects on neuroblastoma prognosis. Lysine methyltransferase 5A (KMT5A), a H4K20me1 methyltransferase, promotes survival and differentiation in neuroblastoma cells by suppressing p53 mediated apoptosis [27]. Overexpression of the DOT1-like histone lysine methyltransferase (DOT1L) histone methytransferase correlates with expression levels of MYCN, solute carrier family 6 member 4 (SLC6A4), and E2F transcription factor 2 (E2F2) genes, triggers the development of neuroblastoma and has been associated with poor prognosis [28]. Histone chaperone chromatin assembly factor 1 subunit A (CHAF1A) promotes advanced-stage neuroblastoma development via H3K9 trimethylation of the survival genes [29]. Lysine demethylase 4B (KDM4B), a lysine demethylase, is responsible for epigenetic regulation of MYCN signaling via histone demethylation in poor prognosis of neuroblastoma [30].

Since the identification of their roles in the pathogenesis of many solid and hematological malignancies, a large proportion of treatment strategies have been targeting epigenetic mechanisms. Because histone acetylation is common in cancer prognosis, investigations focus on HDAC inhibitors, especially. Histone deacetylase 2 (HDAC2) contributes neuroblastoma progression through downregulation of apoptotic miR-183 signaling [31]. The grainyhead-like transcription factor 1 (GRHL1) is suppressed by the promoter hypoacetylation via histone deacetylase 3 (HDAC3) in the advanced-level neuroblastoma [32].

Suppression of CD9 expression in the neuroblastoma by transcriptional activity of histone deacetylase 5 (HDAC5) has been associated with poor prognosis and metastasis [33]. Increased levels of histone deacetylase 8 (HDAC8) expression in neuroblastoma cells have been suggested to play a role in resistance to chemotherapeutics by suppressing the expression of miR-137 and triggering the expression of the ATP binding cassette subfamily B member 1 (MDR1) gene [34]. Upreglation of the SWI/SNF related, matrix associated, actin dependent regulator of chromatin, subfamily A, member 4 (SMARCA4), a chromatin remodeling gene is in the same family with the ATRX, promotes viability of the neuroblastoma cells and it is related to advanced-stage neuroblastoma [35].

As the result of the outputs of the ENCODE project, which was published in 2012, less than 2% of the human genome included protein-coding genes, and large parts of transcriptome composed of pseudogenes and ncRNAs. ncRNAs, which play essential roles both in the regulation of gene expression and in the protein synthesis, contain small RNAs (tRNA, microRNA(miRNA), siRNA, snRNA) and long noncoding RNAs (lnc RNA). miRNAs, single-stranded RNA molecules of about 20 nucleotides and lncRNAs, longer than 200 nucleotides are essential molecules in the gene expression regulation. Since ncRNAs have critical regulatory roles, deregulations are associated with multiplexed pathologies, especially cancers [36].

miRNAs are the basic epigenetic molecules involved in all stages of gene expression regulation. Gene expression has oncogenic (oncomiR) or tumor suppressor properties depending on their regulatory properties.

Members of the miR-17-92 cluster (miR-17-5p, miR-18a, miR-19a, miR-20a, and miR-92) are upregulated with MYCN amplification indicating poor prognosis and treatment resistance via regulation of a main cell cycle regulator cyclin dependent kinase inhibitor 1A (P21) and a apoptotic regulator BCL2-like 11 (BIM) proteins in neuroblastoma cell lines and patients [37, 38]. miR-34a, which is associated with TP53 signaling pathway, acts as a tumor suppressor and downregulates MYCN, E2F transcription factor 3 (E2F3), apoptosis regulator (BCL2), a cell cycle component cyclin D1 (CCND1), and CDK expression. However, in neuroblastoma cells, miR-34a expression is generally silenced with 1p36 deletion [17]. miR-497 is also a tumor suppressor that similarly suppresses the MYCN expression [39]. Upregulation of miR-188-5p and miR-501-5p and downregulation of miR-125b-1 are thought to be associated with chemotherapy resistance [40]. The expression increase of oncomiR miR-221, a negative regulator of the nemo-like kinase (NLK) gene, is characterized by tumor progression and poor prognosis in neuroblastoma cells in relation to MYCN [41]. The low expression of dicer 1, ribonuclease III (DICER), and drosha ribonuclease III (DROSHA) genes, which play a role in the miRNA biogenesis, generally leads to a decrease of miRNA expression in neuroblastoma [42].

Since 2012, lncRNAs have begun to become part of neuroblastoma research, like as the other cancer researches. Studies in this area have focused particularly on the regulation of the expression of genes such as MYCN, ALK, which are highly associated with neuroblastoma pathogenesis, and directing the neuroblastoma cells to apoptotic death. In particular, biomarkers have been identified that indicate a poor prognosis and a high-risk disease group. A cell proliferation regulator Mir-100-Let-7a-2 cluster host gene (MIR100HG) promotes neuroblastoma cell proliferation [43]. lncRNA metastasis associated lung adenocarcinoma transcript 1 (MALAT1) regulates the genes which are responsible for neuronal differentiation, angiogenesis, and migration in neuroblastoma [44–46]. While MYCN upstream transcript (MYCNUT) and small nucleolar RNA host gene 1 (SNHG1) which are associated with high risk, trigger neuroblastoma progression via MYCN amplification, cyclin dependent kinase inhibitor 2A (CAI2), and long intergenic nonprotein coding RNA 467 (LINC00467) promote the neuroblastoma independently of the MYCN expression [47–50]. Downregulation or loss of tumor suppressor lncRNAs cancer susceptibility candidate 15 (CASC15-S) and neuroblastoma associated transcript 1 (NBAT-1), and upregulation of onco-lncRNA ncRAN are associated with advanced-stage neuroblastoma and poor prognosis via increasing cell proliferation and disregulating neuronal differentiation [51–53].

Anti-apoptotic lncRNAs growth arrest specific 5 (GAS5), long intergenic nonprotein coding RNA 1105 (LINC01105) are located in TP53 signaling pathway and regulate apoptosis in neuroblastoma cells. Activation of the lncRNA GAS5, which has two alternative transcripts that both suppress TP53, DNA repair associated (BRCA1) and growth arrest and DNA damage inducible alpha (GADD45A) and stabilize proto-oncogene, E3 ubiquitin protein ligase (MDM2), promotes tumor proliferation in neuroblastoma cells by inhibiting apoptosis and cell cycle arrest [54]. LINC01105 upregulation also suppresses TP53-related apoptosis in neuroblastoma cells. On the other hand, proapoptotic lncRNA maternally expressed 3 (MEG3) is also located TP53 signal pathway and downregulation of MEG3 causes suppression of apoptosis and deregulated differentiation in the neuroblastoma tissues [55]. Even though the epigenetic changes may regulate the prognosis and progression stage in neuroblastoma patients, the knowledge about the regulation mechanisms is still inadequate (**Figure 1**).

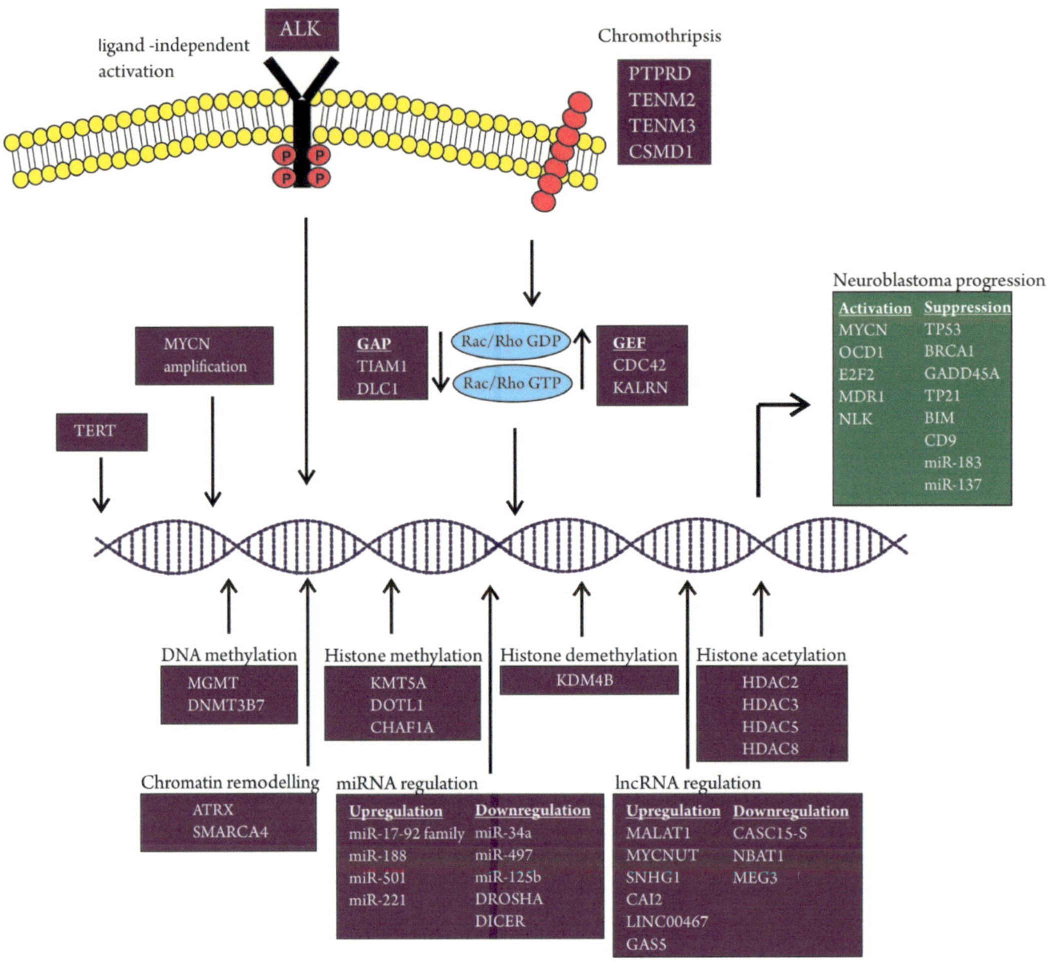

Figure 1. Genetic and epigenetic mechanisms in neuroblastoma.

3. Neuroblastoma stem cell

Neuroblastoma is a heterogeneous cancer and there are many different specific cells in a single tumor. It has been suggested that all types of cancer cells that provide heterogeneous properties are characterized by the differentiation of a single neuroblastoma stem cell [56]. Because cancer stem cells are closely related to both chemotherapy resistance and relapse, the elucidation of the molecular mechanisms of neuroblastoma stem cells is crucial for treatment success.

Neuroblastoma stem cells were first described as I-type cells (intermediate type), malignant cells of neural crest, morphologically located between neuroblastic cells and neural crest cells. I cells are characterized as stem cells because they can produce self-renewal cell lines of two cell types [57].

Polarity loss and asymmetric division of neuronal cells constitute neuroblastoma stem cells during normal neuronal development have been shown in studies conducted in Drosophila melanogaster [58]. Speedy/RINGO cell cycle regulator family member A (SPDYA) regulates the formation of neuroblastoma stem cells by controlling asymmetric division of cells [59]. ALK and MYCN mutations, which have the most important share in the progression of familial and sporadic neuroblastomas, respectively, can constitute neuroblastoma stem cells from neural crest progenitor cells [60]. Repression of TP53 by proto-oncogene, polycomb ring finger (BMI1) causes neuroblastoma induction from embryonic precursors by reducing the response to oncogenic transformation [61]. It is suggested that polo-like kinase 1 (PLK1) expression in neuroblastoma stem cells is one of the factors that contribute to survival and self-renewal [62].

Neuroblastoma stem cells are characterized by upregulation of prominin1 (PROM1/CD133), proto-oncogene receptor tyrosine kinase (KIT/CD117), colony stimulating factor 3 receptor (CSF3R/CD114) cell surface proteins and G protein-coupled receptor class C group 5 member C (GPRC5C), NOTCH1, placental growth factor (PGF), neurotrophic receptor tyrosine kinase 2 (NTRK2), nerve growth factor receptor (NGFR), colony stimulating factor 3 (CSF3), signal transducer and activator of transcription 3 (STAT3), and RB transcriptional corepressor-like 2 (RBL2) genes which play a role in differentiation to malignant neuroblastoma stem cell (**Figure 2**) [63–66].

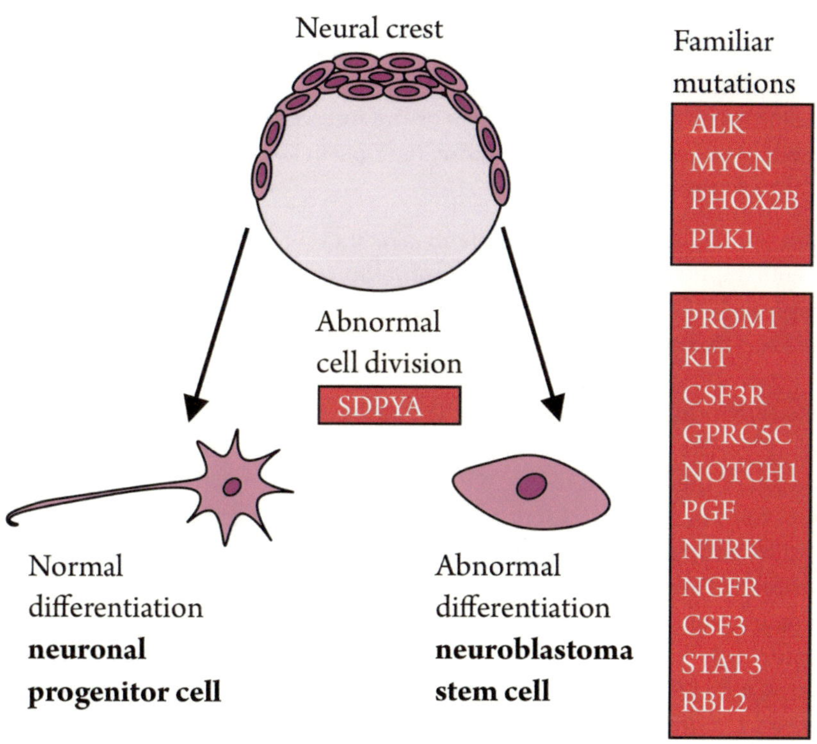

Figure 2. Neurblastoma stem cell.

4. Targeted treatment approach and future perspectives

Retinoic acid, platinum complexes, DNA alkylating agents, and topoisomerase inhibitors are used in the conventional chemotherapy of neuroblastoma. Nevertheless, neuroblastoma cells become resistant to the chemotherapeutics during the time. Mechanisms that cause chemotherapy resistance are frequently associated with MYCN. A novel retinoic acid resistance mechanism includes LIM domain only 4 (LMO4), cytochrome P450 family 26 subfamily A member 1 (CYP26A1), achaete-scute family BHLH transcription factor 1 (ASCL1), ret proto-oncogene (RET), frizzled class receptor 7 (FZD7), and dickkopf WNT signaling pathway inhibitor 1 (DKK1) genes are triggered by MYCN overexpression. These causes may lead to targeting of TGF-β signaling pathway, leading to resistance [67]. MYCN plays a different critical role in resistance to platinum compounds by inhibiting apoptosis through deregulation of PPARG coactivator 1 alpha (PPARGC1A), transcription factor A, mitochondrial (TFAM) genes regulating mitochondrial biogenesis and mitochondrial dynamin-like GTPase (OPA1), mitofusin 2 (MFN2), dynamin 1-like (DRP1) genes regulating mitochondrial dynamics [68]. The identification of resistance mechanisms taking place in different pathways is still ongoing. Most recently, two different resistance formation has been described both calcium metabolism and activation of the hepatocyte growth factor (HGF)/hepatocyte growth factor receptor (MET) signaling pathway [69, 70]. Resistant-dependent or independent relapse also limits the success of conventional chemotherapy.

Conventional chemotherapy resistance and relapse risk have led research to focus on targeted therapy. Currently, targeted treatment approaches aim to induce apoptosis of neuroblastoma cells, dominantly. Moreover, studies of the induction of normal neuronal differentiation, epigenetic regulation, immunotherapy, nanoparticles, and dual mechanisms have been the subject of recent research.

Upregulation of PLK1, the positive regulator of cell cycle and MYCN stabilization, has been associated with high-risk neuroblastoma. Inhibition of PLK1 causes cell cycle arrest and induces apoptosis [71, 72]. Unlike many cancers, TP53 mutations occur less frequently in neuroblastoma. The inhibition of protein phosphatase, Mg^{2+}/Mn^{2+} dependent 1D (PPM1D/Wip1), which is a negative regulator of TP53 mediated cell-death pathway, has been proposed as a novel approach to induce apoptosis through neuroblastoma cells through checkpoint kinase 2 (CHK2)/TP53 [73]. The novel identified proapoptotic brain expressed X-linked (BEX) genes in the downstream of the TP53 signaling pathway are promising as new tumor suppressors by inducing apoptosis in neuroblastoma cells [74]. Inhibition of epidermal growth factor receptor (EGFR) directs neuroblastoma cells to apoptosis through the suppression of the phosphatidylinositol-4,5-bisphosphate 3-kinase (PI3K)/serine/threonine kinase (AKT)/mechanistic target of rapamycin (mTOR) signaling pathway [75]. The inhibition of the G-protein associated receptor tachykinin receptor 1 (TACR1) induces apoptosis and reduces survival in neuroblastoma cells [76]. Targeting the proto-oncogene, nonreceptor tyrosine kinase (SRC)/proto-oncogene 1, nonreceptor tyrosine kinase (ABL) presents a new therapeutic approach by directing neuroblastoma cells to death [77]. Interleukin 24 (IL-24) induces cell death in neuroblastoma via caspase-independent pathway via apoptosis inducing factor (AIF), serine/threonine kinase (ATM), and H2A histone family member X (H2AFX) regulation [78].

Another approach is the induction of normal differentiation of neuroblastoma cells. The ASCL1 gene prevents the neuronal differentiation of neuroblast cells, the main cause of neuroblastoma development, through a mechanism independent of MYCN oncogenes [79]. Coactivation of PPARD regulates cell differentiation, and retinoic acid receptor alpha (RARA), which is involved in conventional therapy, composes a new combinational approach to neuroblastoma therapy by inducing normal differentiation of neuroblasts [80]. Coinhibition of ALK and CDK4/6, Anti-GD2 mAb and HDAC, aurora kinase A (AURKA), and BCL-2, also constitute synergistic approaches to neuroblastoma treatment [81–83].

Epigenetic regulation has great importance in the treatment as well as in the pathogenesis of neuroblastoma. Inhibition of HDAC11 in neuroblastoma suppresses genes associated with proliferation and induces apoptosis. HDAC11 can be seen as a promising goal for treatment [84]. HDAC8 inhibition and miR-137 expression lead to increased chemotherapy sensitivity [34]. miR-497, which regulates the genes associated with proliferation, metastasis, and resistance, is a novel candidate molecule for targeted neuroblastoma therapy [85]. The epigenetic regulator miR-506 suppresses the metastasis of the neuroblastoma cells via inhibiting Rho associated coiled-coil containing protein kinase 1 (ROCK1) which is located in transforming growth factor beta (TGF-B) signaling pathway [86]. Upregulation of ncRNA 45A plays a critical role in tumor proliferation and metastasis by regulating the expression of amyloid beta precursor protein binding family B member 2 (FE65L1), G2, and S-phase expressed 1 (GTSE1) genes [87].

Digestive organ expansion factor (DEF) plays a role in ribosome biogenesis, acts as a regulator in both the development of the peripheral sympathetic nervous system and the development of neuroblastoma. DEF and the other components of the small ribosomal subunit processome involved in ribosome biogenesis have potential use in neuroblastoma targeted therapy [88]. Human ion channel transient receptor potential cation channel subfamily M member 2 (TRPM2), which regulates cell proliferation via mitochondria, is a potential therapeutic target in neuroblastoma [89]. One of the promising approaches in neuroblastoma therapy is to target cell surface proteins such as solute carrier family 6 member 2 (HNET) regulates neurotransmitter homeostasis, ALK, and NTRK2 and neural cell adhesion molecule (NCAM) [90, 91].

It is a promising approach to vaccination through chimeric antigen receptor (CAR)-modified T cells both to create an immunological response to neuroblastoma cells and to increase the level of response [92]. Cancer/testis antigen 1B (CTAG1B) is expressed by various solid tumors including the neuroblastoma, a potential immunotherapy target [93].

Nanoparticles have great potential for the use of diagnosis through fluorescent probes and treatment via encapsulated therapeutic genes (siMyc, siBcl-2, and siVEGF) of neuroblastoma [94]. Targeting drug delivery to neuroblastoma cells may be achieved by genetically engineered biological nanoporus molecules such as diatoms so minimizing damage to healthy cells [95].

Clustered regularly interspaced short palindromic repeats (CRISPRs) and CRISPR-associated protein-9 nuclease (Cas9) systems are valuable targeted genome editing tools that have great potential for molecular medicine applications. The studies aimed to clarify the mechanisms that play a role in pathogenesis and to develop targeted therapies. The activity of aldehyde dehydrogenase 1 (ALDH1) isoenzymes was associated with the aggressive nature of neuroblastoma stem cells in the study using patient-derived xenograft tumors using CRISPR/Cas9 technology [96]. In animal models, DNA methyltransferase 3 alpha (DNMT3a) transactivation using CRISPR/Cas9 technology contributes to the regulation of the methylation of brain cells [97]. Using CRISPR/Cas9 technology, silencing mutant neuroblastoma RAS viral oncogene homolog (NRAS) gene through guide RNAs (gRNAs) in the NRAS-mutant cell line has made cells more sensitive to specific inhibitors [98].

Increased knowledge of neuroblastoma pathology and molecular biology will contribute to the creation of new approaches to diagnosis and treatment and to increased patient life quality and survival rates.

Author details

Bakiye Goker Bagca and Cigir Biray Avci*

*Address all correspondence to: cigir.biray@ege.edu.tr

Department of Medical Biology, Faculty of Medicine, Ege University, Izmir, Turkey

References

[1] Chmielecki J, Bailey M, He J, Elvin J, Vergilio JA, Ramkissoon S, Suh J, Frampton GM, Sun JX, Morley S, Spritz D, Ali S, Gay L, Erlich RL, Ross JS, Buxhaku J, Davies H, Faso V, Germain A, Glanville B, Miller VA, Stephens PJ, Janeway KA, Maris JM, Meshinchi S, Pugh TJ, Shern JF, Lipson D. Genomic profiling of a large set of diverse pediatric cancers identifies known and novel mutations across tumor spectra. Cancer Research. 2017;**77**(2):509-519. DOI: 10.1158/0008-5472.CAN-16-1106

[2] Brodeur GM, Seeger RC, Schwab M, Varmus HE, Bishop JM. Amplification of N-myc in untreated human neuroblastomas correlates with advanced disease stage. Science. 1984;**224**(4653):1121-1124

[3] National Center for Biotechnology Information, U.S. National Library of Medicine. MYCN proto-oncogene, bHLH Transcription Factor [*Homo sapiens* (human)] [Internet]. [Updated: 2017]. Available from: https://www.ncbi.nlm.nih.gov/gene/4613 [Accessed: March 7, 2017]

[4] National Center for Biotechnology Information. MYC proto-oncogene, bHLH Transcription Factor [*Homo sapiens* (human)] [Internet]. [Updated: 2017]. Available from: https://www.ncbi.nlm.nih.gov/gene/4609 [Accessed: March 7, 2017]

[5] Huang M, Weiss WA. Neuroblastoma and MYCN. Cold Spring Harbor Perspectives in Medicine. 2013;**3**(10):a014415. DOI: 10.1101/cshperspect.a014415

[6] Lamant L, Pulford K, Bischof D, Morris SW, Mason DY, Delsol G, Mariamé B. Expression of the ALK tyrosine kinase gene in neuroblastoma. The American Journal of Pathology. 2000;**156**(5):1711-1721. DOI: 10.1016/S0002-9440(10)65042-0

[7] Mossé YP, Laudenslager M, Longo L, Cole KA, Wood A, Attiyeh EF, Laquaglia MJ, Sennett R, Lynch JE, Perri P, Laureys G, Speleman F, Kim C, Hou C, Hakonarson H, Torkamani A, Schork NJ, Brodeur GM, Tonini GP, Rappaport E, Devoto M, Maris JM. Identification of ALK as the major familial neuroblastoma predisposition gene. Nature. 2008;**455**(7215):930-935. DOI: 10.1038/nature07261

[8] Trochet D, Bourdeaut F, Janoueix-Lerosey I, Deville A, de Pontual L, Schleiermacher G, Coze C, Philip N, Frébourg T, Munnich A, Lyonnet S, Delattre O, Amiel J. Germline mutations of the paired-like homeobox 2B (PHOX2B) gene in neuroblastoma. The American Journal of Pathology. 2004;**74**(4):761-764. DOI: 10.1086/383253

[9] Cheung NK, Zhang J, Lu C, Parker M, Bahrami A, Tickoo SK, Heguy A, Pappo AS, Federico S, Dalton J, Cheung IY, Ding L, Fulton R, Wang J, Chen X, Becksfort J, Wu J, Billups CA, Ellison D, Mardis ER, Wilson RK, Downing JR, Dyer MA. Association of age at diagnosis and genetic mutations in patients with neuroblastoma. JAMA. 2012;**307**(10):1062-1071. DOI: 10.1001/jama.2012.228

[10] National Center for Biotechnology Information. ATRX, Chromatin Remodeler [*Homo sapiens* (human)] [Internet]. [Updated: 2017]. Available from: https://www.ncbi.nlm.nih.gov/gene/546 [Accessed: March 7, 2017]

[11] Voon HP, Hughes JR, Rode C, De La Rosa-Velázquez IA, Jenuwein T, Feil R, Higgs DR, Gibbons RJ. ATRX plays a key role in maintaining silencing at interstitial heterochromatic loci and imprinted genes. Cell Reports. 2015;**11**(3):405-418. DOI: 10.1016/j.celrep.2015.03.036

[12] Gunes C, Rudolph KL. The role of telomeres in stem cells and cancer. Cell. 2013;**152**(3) DOI: 10.1016/j.cell.2013.01.010

[13] Heaphy CM, de Wilde RF, Jiao Y, Klein AP, Edil BH, Shi C, Bettegowda C, Rodriguez FJ, Eberhart CG, Hebbar S, Offerhaus GJ, McLendon R, Rasheed BA, He Y, Yan H, Bigner DD, Oba-Shinjo SM, Marie SK, Riggins GJ, Kinzler KW, Vogelstein B, Hruban RH, Maitra A, Papadopoulos N, Meeker AK. Altered telomeres in tumors with ATRX and DAXX mutations. Science. 2011;**333**(6041):425. DOI: 10.1126/science.1207313

[14] Valentijn LJ, Koster J, Zwijnenburg DA, Hasselt NE, van Sluis P, Volckmann R, van Noesel MM, George RE, Tytgat GA, Molenaar JJ, Versteeg R. TERT rearrangements are frequent in neuroblastoma and identify aggressive tumors. Nature Genetics. 2015;**47**(12):1411-1414. DOI: 10.1038/ng.3438

[15] Stephens PJ, Greenman CD, Fu B, Yang F, Bignell GR, Mudie LJ, Pleasance ED, Lau KW, Beare D, Stebbings LA, McLaren S, Lin ML, McBride DJ, Varela I, Nik-Zainal S, Leroy C, Jia M, Menzies A, Butler AP, Teague JW, Quail MA, Burton J, Swerdlow H, Carter NP, Morsberger LA, Iacobuzio-Donahue C, Follows GA, Green AR, Flanagan AM, Stratton MR, Futreal PA, Campbell PJ. Massive genomic rearrangement acquired in a single catastrophic event during cancer development. Cell. 2011;**144**(1):27-40. DOI: 10.1016/j.cell.2010.11.055

[16] Molenaar JJ, Koster J, Zwijnenburg DA, van Sluis P, Valentijn LJ, van der Ploeg I, Hamdi M, van Nes J, Westerman BA, van Arkel J, Ebus ME, Haneveld F, Lakeman A, Schild L,

Molenaar P, Stroeken P, van Noesel MM, Ora I, Santo EE, Caron HN, Westerhout EM, Versteeg R. Sequencing of neuroblastoma identifies chromothripsis and defects in neuritogenesis genes. Nature. 2012;**483**(7391):589-593. DOI: 10.1038/nature10910

[17] Henrich KO, Schwab M, Westermann F. 1p36 tumor suppression—A matter of dosage? Cancer Research. 2012;**72**(23):6079-6088. DOI: 10.1158/0008-5472.CAN-12-2230

[18] Bown N, Cotterill S, Lastowska M, O'Neill S, Pearson AD, Plantaz D, Meddeb M, Danglot G, Brinkschmidt C, Christiansen H, Laureys G, Speleman F, Nicholson J, Bernheim A, Betts DR, Vandesompele J, Van Roy N. Gain of chromosome arm 17q and adverse outcome in patients with neuroblastoma. The New England Journal of Medicine. 1999;**340**(25):1954-1961

[19] Bosse KR, Maris JM. Advances in the translational genomics of neuroblastoma: From improving risk stratification and revealing novel biology to identifying actionable genomic alterations. Cancer. 2016;**122**(1):20-33. DOI: DOI: 10.1002/cncr.29706

[20] Oldridge DA, Wood AC, Weichert-Leahey N, Crimmins I, Sussman R, Winter C, McDaniel LD, Diamond M, Hart LS, Zhu S, Durbin AD, Abraham BJ, Anders L, Tian L, Zhang S, Wei JS, Khan J, Bramlett K, Rahman N, Capasso M, Iolascon A, Gerhard DS, Guidry Auvil JM, Young RA, Hakonarson H, Diskin SJ, Look AT, Maris JM. Genetic predisposition to neuroblastoma mediated by a LMO1 super-enhancer polymorphism. Nature. 2015;**528**(7582):418-421. DOI: 10.1038/nature15540

[21] Diskin SJ, Capasso M, Diamond M, Oldridge DA, Conkrite K, Bosse KR, Russell MR, Iolascon A, Hakonarson H, Devoto M, Maris JM. Rare variants in TP53 and susceptibility to neuroblastoma. Journal of the National Cancer Institute. 2014;**106**(4):dju047. DOI: 10.1093/jnci/dju047

[22] Bird A. Perceptions of epigenetics. Nature. 2007;**447**(7143):396-398. DOI: 10.1038/nature 05913

[23] Mayol G, Martín-Subero JI, Ríos J, Queiros A, Kulis M, Suñol M, Esteller M, Gómez S, Garcia I, de Torres C, Rodríguez E, Galván P, Mora J, Lavarino C. DNA hypomethylation affects cancer-related biological functions and genes relevant in neuroblastoma pathogenesis. PLoS One. 2012;**7**(11):e48401. DOI: 10.1371/journal.pone.0048401

[24] Decock A, Ongenaert M, Hoebeeck J, De Preter K, Van Peer G, Van Criekinge W, Ladenstein R, Schulte JH, Noguera R, Stallings RL, Van Damme A, Laureys G, Vermeulen J, Van Maerken T, Speleman F, Vandesompele J. Genome-wide promoter methylation analysis in neuroblastoma identifies prognostic methylation biomarkers. Genome Biology. 2012;**13**(10):R95. DOI: 10.1186/gb-2012-13-10-r95

[25] Wickström M, Dyberg C, Milosevic J, Einvik C, Calero R, Sveinbjörnsson B, Sandén E, Darabi A, Siesjö P, Kool M, Kogner P, Baryawno N, Johnsen JI. Wnt/β-catenin pathway regulates MGMT gene expression in cancer and inhibition of Wnt signalling prevents chemoresistance. Nature Communications. 2015;**6**:8904. DOI: 10.1038/ncomms9904

[26] Ostler KR, Yang Q, Looney TJ, Zhang L, Vasanthakumar A, Tian Y, Kocherginsky M, Raimondi SL, DeMaio JG, Salwen HR, Gu S, Chlenski A, Naranjo A, Gill A, Peddinti

R, Lahn BT, Cohn SL, Godley LA. Truncated DNMT3B isoform DNMT3B7 suppresses growth, induces differentiation, and alters DNA methylation in human neuroblastoma. Cancer Research. 2012;**72**(18):4714-4723. DOI: 10.1158/0008-5472.CAN-12-0886

[27] Veschi V, Liu Z, Voss TC, Ozbun L, Gryder B, Yan C, Hu Y, Ma A, Jin J, Mazur SJ, Lam N, Souza BK, Giannini G, Hager GL, Arrowsmith CH, Khan J, Appella E, Thiele CJ. Epigenetic siRNA and chemical screens identify SETD8 inhibition as a therapeutic strategy for p53 activation in High-Risk neuroblastoma. Cancer Cell. 2017;**31**(1):50-63. DOI: 10.1016/j.ccell.2016.12.002

[28] Wong M, Tee AE, Milazzo G, Bell JL, Poulos RC, Atmadibrata B, Sun Y, Jing D, Ho N, Ling D, Liu PY, Zhang XD, Hüttelmaier S, Wong JW, Wang J, Polly P, Perini G, Scarlett CJ, Liu T. The histone methyltransferase DOT1L promotes neuroblastoma by regulating gene transcription. Cancer Res. 2017 May 1;**77**(9):2522-2533. doi: 10.1158/0008-5472.CAN-16-1663.

[29] Barbieri E, De Preter K, Capasso M, Chen Z, Hsu DM, Tonini GP, Lefever S, Hicks J, Versteeg R, Pession A, Speleman F, Kim ES, Shohet JM. Histone chaperone CHAF1A inhibits differentiation and promotes aggressive neuroblastoma. Cancer Research. 2014;**74**(3):765-774. DOI: 10.1158/0008-5472.CAN-13-1315

[30] Yang J, AlTahan AM, Hu D, Wang Y, Cheng PH, Morton CL, Qu C, Nathwani AC, Shohet JM, Fotsis T, Koster J, Versteeg R, Okada H, Harris AL, Davidoff AM. The role of histone demethylase KDM4B in Myc signaling in neuroblastoma. Journal of the National Cancer Institute. 2015;**107**(6):djv080. DOI: 10.1093/jnci/djv080

[31] Lodrini M, Oehme I, Schroeder C, Milde T, Schier MC, Kopp-Schneider A, Schulte JH, Fischer M, De Preter K, Pattyn F, Castoldi M, Muckenthaler MU, Kulozik AE, Westermann F, Witt O, Deubzer HE. MYCN and HDAC2 cooperate to repress miR-183 signaling in neuroblastoma. Nucleic Acids Research. 2013;**41**(12):6018-6033. DOI: 10.1093/nar/gkt346

[32] Fabian J, Lodrini M, Oehme I, Schier MC, Thole TM, Hielscher T, Kopp-Schneider A, Opitz L, Capper D, von Deimling A, Wiegand I, Milde T, Mahlknecht U, Westermann F, Popanda O, Roels F, Hero B, Berthold F, Fischer M, Kulozik AE, Witt O, Deubzer HE. GRHL1 acts as tumor suppressor in neuroblastoma and is negatively regulated by MYCN and HDAC3. Cancer Research. 2014;**74**(9):2604-2616. DOI: 10.1158/0008-5472.CAN-13-1904

[33] Fabian J, Opitz D, Althoff K, Lodrini M, Hero B, Volland R, Beckers A, de Preter K, Decock A, Patil N, Abba M, Kopp-Schneider A, Astrahantseff K, Wünschel J, Pfeil S, Ercu M, Künkele A, Hu J, Thole T, Schweizer L, Mechtersheimer G, Carter D, Cheung BB, Popanda O, von Deimling A, Koster J, Versteeg R, Schwab M, Marshall GM, Speleman F, Erb U, Zoeller M, Allgayer H, Simon T, Fischer M, Kulozik AE, Eggert A, Witt O, Schulte JH, Deubzer HE. MYCN and HDAC5 transcriptionally repress CD9 to trigger invasion and metastasis in neuroblastoma. Oncotarget. 2016;**7**(41):66344-66359. DOI: 10.18632/oncotarget.11662

[34] Zhao G, Wang G, Bai H, Li T, Gong F, Yang H, Wen J, Wang W. Targeted inhibition of HDAC8 increases the doxorubicin sensitivity of neuroblastoma cells via up regulation of miR-137. European Journal of Pharmacology. 2017;**802**:20-26. DOI: 10.1016/j.ejphar.2017.02.035

[35] Jubierre L, Soriano A, Planells-Ferrer L, París-Coderch L, Tenbaum SP, Romero OA, Moubarak RS, Almazán-Moga A, Molist C, Roma J, Navarro S, Noguera R, Sánchez-Céspedes M, Comella JX, Palmer HG, Sánchez de Toledo J, Gallego S, Segura MF. BRG1/SMARCA4 is essential for neuroblastoma cell viability through modulation of cell death and survival pathways. Oncogene. 2016;**35**(39):5179-5190. DOI: 10.1038/onc.2016.50

[36] The ENCODE Project Consortium. An integrated encyclopedia of DNA elements in the human genome. Nature. 2012;**489**(7414):57-74. DOI: 10.1038/nature11247

[37] Chen Y, Stallings RL. Differential patterns of microRNA expression in neuroblastoma are correlated with prognosis, differentiation, and apoptosis. Cancer Research. 2007;**67**(3):976-983. DOI: 10.1158/0008-5472.CAN-06-3667

[38] Fontana L, Fiori ME, Albini S, Cifaldi L, Giovinazzi S, Forloni M, Boldrini R, Donfrancesco A, Federici V, Giacomini P, Peschle C, Fruci D. Antagomir-17-5p abolishes the growth of therapy-resistant neuroblastoma through p21 and BIM. PLoS One. 2008;**3**(5):e2236. DOI: 10.1371/journal.pone.0002236

[39] Creevey L, Ryan J, Harvey H, Bray IM, Meehan M, Khan AR, Stallings RL. MicroRNA-497 increases apoptosis in MYCN amplified neuroblastoma cells by targeting the key cell cycle regulator WEE1. Molecular Cancer. 2013;**12**:23. DOI: 10.1186/1476-4598-12-23

[40] Ayers D, Mestdagh P, Van Maerken T, Vandesompele J. Identification of miRNAs contributing to neuroblastoma chemoresistance. Computational and Structural Biotechnology. 2015;**13**:307-319. DOI: 10.1016/j.csbj.2015.04.003

[41] He XY, Tan ZL, Mou Q, Liu FJ, Liu S, Yu CW, Zhu J, Lv LY, Zhang J, Wang S, Bao L, Peng B, Zhao H, Zou L. MicroRNA-221 enhances MYCN via targeting nemo-like kinase, and functions as an oncogene related to poor prognosis in neuroblastoma. Clin Cancer Res. 2016. Jan 16;1-14. DOI: 10.1158/1078-0432.CCR-16-1591

[42] Lin RJ, Lin YC, Chen J, Kuo HH, Chen YY, Diccianni MB, London WB, Chang CH, Yu AL. MicroRNA signature and expression of Dicer and Drosha can predict prognosis and delineate risk groups in neuroblastoma. Cancer Research. 2010;**70**(20):7841-7850. DOI: 10.1158/0008-5472.CAN-10-0970

[43] Bevilacqua V, Gioia U, Di Carlo V, Tortorelli AF, Colombo T, Bozzoni I, Laneve P, Caffarelli E. Identification of linc-NeD125, a novel long noncoding RNA that hosts miR-125b-1 and negatively controls proliferation of human neuroblastoma cells. RNA Biology. 2015;**12**(12):1323-1337. DOI: 10.1080/15476286.2015.1096488

[44] Chen L, Feng P, Zhu X, He S, Duan J, Zhou D. Long non-coding RNA Malat1 promotes neurite outgrowth through activation of ERK/MAPK signalling pathway in N2a cells. Journal of Cellular and Molecular Medicine. 2016;**20**(11):2102-2110. DOI: 10.1111/jcmm.12904

[45] . Tee AE, Liu B, Song R, Li J, Pasquier E, Cheung BB, Jiang C, Marshall GM, Haber M, Norris MD, Fletcher JI, Dinger ME, Liu T. The long noncoding RNA MALAT1 promotes tumor-driven angiogenesis by up-regulating pro-angiogenic gene expression. Oncotarget. 2016;**7**(8):8663-8675. DOI: 10.18632/oncotarget.6675

[46] Tee AE, Ling D, Nelson C, Atmadibrata B, Dinger ME, Xu N, Mizukami T, Liu PY, Liu B, Cheung B, Pasquier E, Haber M, Norris MD, Suzuki T, Marshall GM, Liu T. The histone demethylase JMJD1A induces cell migration and invasion by up-regulating the expression of the long noncoding RNA MALAT1. Oncotarget. 2014;**5**(7):1793-1804

[47] Liu PY, Erriquez D, Marshall GM, Tee AE, Polly P, Wong M, Liu B, Bell JL, Zhang XD, Milazzo G, Cheung BB, Fox A, Swarbrick A, Hüttelmaier S, Kavallaris M, Perini G, Mattick JS, Dinger ME, Liu T. Effects of a novel long noncoding RNA, lncUSMycN, on N-Myc expression and neuroblastoma progression. J Natl Cancer Inst. 2014 Jun 6;**106**(7). pii: dju113. doi: 10.1093/jnci/dju113. DOI: 10.1093/jnci/dju359

[48] Sahu D, Hsu CL, Lin CC, Yang TW, Hsu WM, Ho SY, Juan HF, Huang HC. Co-expression analysis identifies long noncoding RNA SNHG1 as a novel predictor for event-free survival in neuroblastoma. Oncotarget. 2016;**7**(36):58022-58037. DOI: 10.18632/oncotarget.11158

[49] Barnhill LM, Williams RT, Cohen O, Kim Y, Batova A, Mielke JA, Messer K, Pu M, Bao L, Yu AL, Diccianni MB. High expression of CAI2, a 9p21-embedded long noncoding RNA, contributes to advanced-stage neuroblastoma. Cancer Research. 2014;**74**(14):3753-3763. DOI: 10.1158/0008-5472.CAN-13-3447

[50] Atmadibrata B, Liu PY, Sokolowski N, Zhang L, Wong M, Tee AE, Marshall GM, Liu T. The novel long noncoding RNA linc00467 promotes cell survival but is down-regulated by N-Myc. PLoS One. 2014;**9**(2):e88112. DOI: 10.1371/journal.pone.0088112

[51] Russell MR, Penikis A, Oldridge DA, Alvarez-Dominguez JR, McDaniel L, Diamond M, Padovan O, Raman P, Li Y, Wei JS, Zhang S, Gnanchandran J, Seeger R, Asgharzadeh S, Khan J, Diskin SJ, Maris JM, Cole KA. CASC15-S is a tumor suppressor lncRNA at the 6p22 neuroblastoma susceptibility locus. Cancer Research. 2015;**75**(15):3155-3166. DOI: 10.1158/0008-5472.CAN-14-3613

[52] Yu M, Ohira M, Li Y, Niizuma H, Oo ML, Zhu Y, Ozaki T, Isogai E, Nakamura Y, Koda T, Oba S, Yu B, Nakagawara A. High expression of ncRAN, a novel non-coding RNA mapped to chromosome 17q25.1, is associated with poor prognosis in neuroblastoma. International Journal of Oncology. 2009;**34**(4):931-938

[53] Pandey GK, Mitra S, Subhash S, Hertwig F, Kanduri M, Mishra K, Fransson S, Ganeshram A, Mondal T, Bandaru S, Ostensson M, Akyürek LM, Abrahamsson J, Pfeifer S, Larsson E, Shi L, Peng Z, Fischer M, Martinsson T, Hedborg F, Kogner P, Kanduri C. The risk-associated long noncoding RNA NBAT-1 controls neuroblastoma progression by regulating cell proliferation and neuronal differentiation. Cancer Cell. 2014;**26**(5):722-737. DOI: 10.1016/j.ccell.2014.09.014

[54] Mazar J, Rosado A, Shelley J, Marchica J, Westmoreland TJ. The long non-coding RNA GAS5 differentially regulates cell cycle arrest and apoptosis through activation of BRCA1 and p53 in human neuroblastoma. Oncotarget. 2017;**8**(4):6589-6607. DOI: 10.18632/oncotarget.14244

[55] Tang W, Dong K, Li K, Dong R, Zheng S. MEG3, HCN3 and linc01105 influence the proliferation and apoptosis of neuroblastoma cells via the HIF-1α and p53 pathways. Scientific Reports. 2016;**6**:36268. DOI: 10.1038/srep36268

[56] Walton JD, Kattan DR, Thomas SK, Spengler BA, Guo HF, Biedler JL, Cheung NK, Ross RA. Characteristics of stem cells from human neuroblastoma cell lines and in tumors. Neoplasia. 2004;**6**(6):838-845

[57] Ross RA, Spengler BA, Domènech C, Porubcin M, Rettig WJ, Biedler JL. Neuroblastoma stem cells were first described as I-type cells (intermediate type), malignant cells of neural crest, morphologically located between neuroblastic cells and neural crest cells. I cells are characterized as stem cells because they can produce multi-potent and self-renewal cell lines of two cell types. Cell Growth & Differentiation. 1995;**6**(4):449-456

[58] Caussinus E, Gonzalez C. Induction of tumor growth by altered stem-cell asymmetric division in Drosophila melanogaster. Nature Genetics. 2005;**37**(10):1125-1129

[59] Lubanska D, Porter LA. The atypical cell cycle regulator Spy1 suppresses differentiation of the neuroblastoma stem cell population. Oncoscience. 2014;**1**(5):336-348

[60] Schulte JH, Lindner S, Bohrer A, Maurer J, De Preter K, Lefever S, Heukamp L, Schulte S, Molenaar J, Versteeg R, Thor T, Künkele A, Vandesompele J, Speleman F, Schorle H, Eggert A, Schramm A. MYCN and ALKF1174L are sufficient to drive neuroblastoma development from neural crest progenitor cells. Oncogene. 2013;**32**(8):1059-1065. DOI: 10.1038/onc.2012.106

[61] Calao M, Sekyere EO, Cui HJ, Cheung BB, Thomas WD, Keating J, Chen JB, Raif A, Jankowski K, Davies NP, Bekkum MV, Chen B, Tan O, Ellis T, Norris MD, Haber M, Kim ES, Shohet JM, Trahair TN, Liu T, Wainwright BJ, Ding HF, Marshall GM. Direct effects of Bmi1 on p53 protein stability inactivates oncoprotein stress responses in embryonal cancer precursor cells at tumor initiation. Oncogene. 2013;**32**(31):3616-3626. DOI: 10.1038/onc.2012.368

[62] Grinshtein N, Datti A, Fujitani M, Uehling D, Prakesch M, Isaac M, Irwin MS, Wrana JL, Al-Awar R, Kaplan DR. Small molecule kinase inhibitor screen identifies polo-like kinase 1 as a target for neuroblastoma tumor-initiating cells. Cancer Research. 2011;**71**(4):1385-1395. DOI: 10.1158/0008-5472.CAN-10-2484

[63] Zage PE, Whittle SB, Shohet JM. CD114: A new member of the neural Crest-Derived cancer stem cell marker family. Journal of Cellular Biochemistry. 2017;**118**(2):221-231. DOI: 10.1002/jcb.25656

[64] Ross RA, Walton JD, Han D, Guo HF, Cheung NK. A distinct gene expression signature characterizes human neuroblastoma cancer stem cells. Stem Cell Research. 2015;**15**(2):419-426. DOI: 10.1016/j.scr.2015.08.008

[65] Agarwal S, Lakoma A, Chen Z, Hicks J, Metelitsa LS, Kim ES, Shohet JM. G-CSF promotes neuroblastoma tumorigenicity and metastasis via STAT3-Dependent cancer stem cell activation. Cancer Research. 2015;**75**(12):2566-2579. DOI: 10.1158/0008-5472.CAN-14-2946

[66] Jori FP, Galderisi U, Piegari E, Peluso G, Cipollaro M, Cascino A, Giordano A, Melone MA. RB2/p130 ectopic gene expression in neuroblastoma stem cells: Evidence of cell-fate restriction and induction of differentiation. Biochemical Journal. 2001;**360**(Pt 3):569-577

[67] Duffy DJ, Krstic A, Halasz M, Schwarzl T, Konietzny A, Iljin K, Higgins DG, Kolch W. Retinoic acid and TGF-β signalling cooperate to overcome MYCN-induced retinoid resistance. Genome Medicine. 2017;**9**(1):15. DOI: 10.1186/s13073-017-0407-3

[68] Casinelli G, LaRosa J, Sharma M, Cherok E, Banerjee S, Branca M, Edmunds L, Wang Y, Sims-Lucas S, Churley L, Kelly S, Sun M, Stolz D, Graves JA. N-Myc overexpression increases cisplatin resistance in neuroblastoma via deregulation of mitochondrial dynamics. Cell Death Discovery. 2016;**2**:16082. DOI: 10.1038/cddiscovery.2016.82

[69] Florea AM, Varghese E, McCallum JE, Mahgoub S, Helmy I, Varghese S, Gopinath N, Sass S, Theis FJ, Reifenberger G, Büsselberg D. Calcium-regulatory proteins as modulators of chemotherapy in human neuroblastoma. Oncotarget. 2017;**8**(14):22876-22893. DOI: 10.18632/oncotarget.15283

[70] Daudigeos-Dubus E, Le Dret L, Bawa O, Opolon P, Vievard A, Villa I, Bosq J, Vassal G, Geoerger B. Dual inhibition using cabozantinib overcomes HGF/MET signaling mediated resistance to pan-VEGFR inhibition in orthotopic and metastatic neuroblastoma tumors. International Journal of Oncology. 2017;**50**(1):203-211. DOI: 10.3892/ijo.2016.3792

[71] Pajtler KW, Sadowski N, Ackermann S, Althoff K, Schönbeck K, Batzke K, Schäfers S, Odersky A, Heukamp L, Astrahantseff K, Künkele A, Deubzer HE, Schramm A, Sprüssel A, Thor T, Lindner S, Eggert A, Fischer M, Schulte JH. The GSK461364 PLK1 inhibitor exhibits strong antitumoral activity in preclinical neuroblastoma models. Oncotarget. 2017;**8**(4):6730-6741. DOI: 10.18632/oncotarget.14268

[72] Xiao D, Yue M, Su H, Ren P, Jiang J, Li F, Hu Y, Du H, Liu H, Qing G. Polo-like Kinase-1 regulates myc stabilization and activates a feedforward circuit promoting tumor cell survival. Molecular Cell. 2016;**64**(3):493-506. DOI: 10.1016/j.molcel.2016.09.016

[73] Chen Z, Wang L, Yao D, Yang T, Cao WM, Dou J, Pang JC, Guan S, Zhang H, Yu Y, Zhao Y, Wang Y, Xu X, Shi Y, Patel R, Zhang H, Vasudevan SA, Liu S, Yang J, Nuchtern JG. Wip1 inhibitor GSK2830371 inhibits neuroblastoma growth by inducing Chk2/p53-mediated apoptosis. Scientific Reports. 2016;**6**:38011. DOI: 10.1038/srep38011

[74] Sidhar H, Giri RK. Induction of Bex genes by curcumin is associated with apoptosis and activation of p53 in N2a neuroblastoma cells. Scientific Reports. 2017;**7**:41420. DOI: 10.1038/srep41420

[75] Mao X, Chen Z, Zhao Y, Yu Y, Guan S, Woodfield SE, Vasudevan SA, Tao L, Pang JC, Lu J, Zhang H, Zhang F, Yang J. Novel multi-targeted ErbB family inhibitor afatinib blocks EGF-induced signaling and induces apoptosis in neuroblastoma. Oncotarget. 2017;**8**(1):1555-1568. DOI: 10.18632/oncotarget.13657

[76] Henssen AG, Odersky A, Szymansky A, Seiler M, Althoff K, Beckers A, Speleman F, Schäfers S, De Preter K, Astrahanseff K, Struck J, Schramm A, Eggert A, Bergmann A, Schulte JH. Targeting tachykinin receptors in neuroblastoma. Oncotarget. 2017;**8**(1):430-443. DOI: 10.18632/oncotarget.1344

[77] Bieerkehazhi S, Chen Z, Zhao Y, Yu Y, Zhang H, Vasudevan SA, Woodfield SE, Tao L, Yi JS, Muscal JA, Pang JC, Guan S, Zhang H, Nuchtern JG, Li H, Li H, Yang J. Novel Src/Abl tyrosine kinase inhibitor bosutinib suppresses neuroblastoma growth via inhibiting Src/Abl signaling. Oncotarget. 2017;**8**(1):1469-1480. DOI: 10.18632/oncotarget.13643

[78] Bhoopathi P, Lee N, Pradhan AK, Shen XN, Das SK, Sarkar D, Emdad L, Fisher PB. mda-7/IL-24 induces cell death in neuroblastoma through a novel mechanism involving AIF and ATM. Cancer Research. 2016;**76**(12):3572-3582. DOI: 10.1158/0008-5472.CAN-15-2959

[79] Kasim M, Heß V, Scholz H, Persson PB, Fähling M. Achaete-Scute homolog 1 expression controls cellular differentiation of neuroblastoma. Frontiers in Molecular Neuroscience. 2016;**9**:156. DOI: 10.3389/fnmol.2016.00156

[80] Yao PL, Chen L, Dobrzański TP, Zhu B, Kang BH, Müller R, Gonzalez FJ, Peters JM. Peroxisome proliferator-activated receptor-β/δ inhibits human neuroblastoma cell tumorigenesis by inducing p53- and SOX2-mediated cell differentiation. Molecular Carcinogenesis. 2016;**56**(5):1472-1483. DOI: 10.1002/mc.22607

[81] Wood A, Krytska K, Ryles HT, Infarinato NR, Sano R, Hansel TD, Hart LS, King F, Smith TR, Ainscow E, Grandinetti KB, Tuntland T, Kim S, Caponigro G, He YQ, Krupa S, Li N, Harris J, Mosse YP. Dual ALK and CDK4/6 inhibition demonstrates on-target synergy against neuroblastoma. Clin Cancer Res. 2016. Dec 16;1-13. DOI: 10.1158/1078-0432.CCR-16-1114

[82] Kroesen M, Büll C, Gielen PR, Brok IC, Armandari I, Wassink M, Looman MW, Boon L, den Brok MH, Hoogerbrugge PM, Adema GJ. Anti-GD2 mAb and Vorinostat synergize in the treatment of neuroblastoma. Oncoimmunology. 2016;**5**(6):e1164919. DOI: 10.1080/2162402X.2016.1164919

[83] Ham J, Costa C, Sano R, Lochmann TL, Sennott EM, Patel NU, Dastur A, Gomez-Caraballo M, Krytska K, Hata AN, Floros KV, Hughes MT, Jakubik CT, Heisey DA, Ferrell JT, Bristol ML, March RJ, Yates C, Hicks MA, Nakajima W, Gowda M, Windle BE, Dozmorov MG, Garnett MJ, McDermott U, Harada H, Taylor SM, Morgan IM, Benes CH, Engelman JA, Mossé YP, Faber AC. Exploitation of the Apoptosis-Primed state of MYCN-Amplified neuroblastoma to develop a potent and specific targeted therapy combination. Cancer Cell. 2016;**29**(2):159-172. DOI: 10.1016/j.ccell.2016.01.002

[84] Thole TM, Lodrini M, Fabian J, Wuenschel J, Pfeil S, Hielscher T, Kopp-Schneider A, Heinicke U, Fulda S, Witt O, Eggert A, Fischer M, Deubzer HE. Neuroblastoma cells depend on HDAC11 for mitotic cell cycle progression and survival. Cell Death & Disease. 2017;**8**(3):e2635. DOI: 10.1038/cddis.2017.49

[85] Soriano A, París-Coderch L, Jubierre L, Martínez A, Zhou X, Piskareva O, Bray I, Vidal I, Almazán-Moga A, Molist C, Roma J, Bayascas JR, Casanovas O, Stallings RL, Sánchez de Toledo J, Gallego S, Segura MF. MicroRNA-497 impairs the growth of chemoresistant neuroblastoma cells by targeting cell cycle, survival and vascular permeability genes. Oncotarget. 2016;**7**(8):9271-9287. DOI: 10.18632/oncotarget.7005

[86] Li D, Cao Y, Li J, Xu J, Liu Q, Sun X. miR-506 suppresses neuroblastoma metastasis by targeting ROCK1. Oncology Letters. 2017;**13**(1):417-422. DOI: 10.3892/ol.2016.5442

[87] Penna I, Gigoni A, Costa D, Vella S, Russo D, Poggi A, Villa F, Brizzolara A, Canale C, Mescola A, Daga A, Russo C, Nizzari M, Florio T, Menichini P, Pagano A. The inhibition of 45A ncRNA expression reduces tumor formation, affecting tumor nodules compactness and metastatic potential in neuroblastoma cells. Oncotarget. 2017;**8**(5):8189-8205. DOI: 10.18632/oncotarget.14138

[88] Tao T, Sondalle SB, Shi H, Zhu S, Perez-Atayde AR, Peng J, Baserga SJ, Look AT. The pre-rRNA processing factor DEF is rate limiting for the pathogenesis of MYCN-driven neuroblastoma. Oncogene. 2017 Mar; 1-16. DOI: 10.1038/onc.2016.527

[89] Bao L, Chen SJ, Conrad K, Keefer K, Abraham T, Lee JP, Wang J, Zhang XQ, Hirschler-Laszkiewicz I, Wang HG, Dovat S, Gans B, Madesh M, Cheung JY, Miller BA. Depletion of the human Ion channel TRPM2 in neuroblastoma demonstrates its key role in cell survival through modulation of mitochondrial reactive oxygen species and bioenergetics. Journal of Biological Chemistry. 2016;**291**(47):24449-24464

[90] Haddad Y, Heger Z, Adam V. Targeting neuroblastoma cell surface proteins: Recommendations for homology modeling of hNET, ALK, and TrkB. Frontiers in Molecular Neuroscience. 2017;**10**:7. DOI: 10.3389/fnmol.2017.00007

[91] Markovsky E, Eldar-Boock A, Ben-Shushan D, Baabur-Cohen H, Yeini E, Pisarevsky E, Many A, Aviel-Ronen S, Barshack I, Satchi-Fainaro R. Targeting NCAM-expressing neuroblastoma with polymeric precision nanomedicine. Journal of Controlled Release. 2017;**249**:162-172. DOI: 10.1016/j.jconrel.2017.01.044

[92] Tanaka M, Tashiro H, Omer B, Lapteva N, Ando J, Ngo M, Mehta B, Dotti G, Kinchington PR, Leen AM, Rossig C, Rooney CM. Vaccination targeting native receptors to enhance the function and proliferation of chimeric antigen receptor (CAR)-modified T cells. Clin Cancer Res. 2017 Feb 9;1-11. DOI: 10.1158/1078-0432.CCR-16-2138

[93] Singh N, Kulikovskaya I, Barrett DM, Binder-Scholl G, Jakobsen B, Martinez D, Pawel B, June CH, Kalos MD, Grupp SA. T cells targeting NY-ESO-1 demonstrate efficacy against disseminated neuroblastoma. Oncoimmunology. 2015;**5**(1):e1040216

[94] Lee J, Jeong EJ, Lee YK, Kim K, Kwon IC, Lee KY. Optical imaging and gene therapy with Neuroblastoma-Targeting polymeric nanoparticles for potential theranostic applications. Small. 2016;**12**(9):1201-1211. DOI: 10.1002/smll.201501913

[95] Delalat B, Sheppard VC, Rasi Ghaemi S, Rao S, Prestidge CA, McPhee G, Rogers ML, Donoghue JF, Pillay V, Johns TG, Kröger N, Voelcker NH. Targeted drug delivery using genetically engineered diatom biosilica. Nature Communications. 2015;**6**:8791. DOI: 10.1038/ncomms9791

[96] Flahaut M, Jauquier N, Chevalier N, Nardou K, Balmas Bourloud K, Joseph JM, Barras D, Widmann C, Gross N, Renella R, Mühlethaler-Mottet A. Aldehyde dehydrogenase activity plays a Key role in the aggressive phenotype of neuroblastoma. BMC Cancer. 2016;**16**(1):781

[97] Kyono Y, Subramani A, Ramadoss P, Hollenberg AN, Bonett RM, Denver RJ. Liganded thyroid hormone receptors transactivate the DNA methyltransferase 3a gene in mouse neuronal cells. Endocrinology. 2016;**157**(9):3647-3657. DOI: 10.1210/en.2015-1529

[98] Kiessling MK, Schuierer S, Stertz S, Beibel M, Bergling S, Knehr J, Carbone W, de Vallière C, Tchinda J, Bouwmeester T, Seuwen K, Rogler G, Roma G. Identification of oncogenic driver mutations by genome-wide CRISPR-Cas9 dropout screening. BMC Genomics. 2016;**17**(1):723. DOI: 10.1186/s12864-016-3042-2

Chapter 6

Telomeres and Telomerase in Neuroblastoma

Joëlle El Hajj, Delphine Garsuault, Claire Bouyer,
Eric Nguyen, George Hilal and
Evelyne Ségal-Bendirdjian

Additional information is available at the end of the chapter

http://dx.doi.org/10.5772/intechopen.69567

Abstract

Telomeres are nucleoprotein structures located at the ends of linear chromosomes. In most human adult normal somatic cells, telomeres shorten after each cellular division. This shortening ultimately leads to senescence and/or apoptosis. By contrast, in most cancer cells, telomerase activation compensates this loss and confers to these cells their infinite cell proliferation potential. Neuroblastoma (NBL) is a malignant tumor of the peripheral sympathetic nervous system and the most frequent extracranial solid tumor of childhood. NBLs are remarkably heterogeneous both at the levels of biology, genetic and clinical courses. Indeed, some of NBLs can regress spontaneously or after a mild treatment, while others are in the high-risk category with poor prognosis. The molecular bases underlying this heterogeneity are poorly understood. MYCN (V-Myc Avian Myelocytomatosis Viral Oncogene Neuroblastoma-derived Homolog) amplification, recognized as strongly associated with unfavorable patient outcome, is found in only 40% of the high-risk disease, indicating the involvement of other mechanisms. Recent observations suggest that telomerase expression and telomere dysfunctions may be one critical step in NBL development. This review provides recent insights on telomeres/telomerase regulation in NBL. Because of their involvement in the tumor cell biology, telomere and telomerase are currently at the core of new drug development.

Keywords: telomerase, telomeres, regulation, therapies, neuroblastoma

1. Introduction

Cancer development is a multistep process requiring genetic and epigenetic events leading to the deregulation of the expression of key genes. Among these genes, telomerase, by its

INTECH
open science | open minds

© 2017 The Author(s). Licensee InTech. This chapter is distributed under the terms of the Creative Commons Attribution License (http://creativecommons.org/licenses/by/3.0), which permits unrestricted use, distribution, and reproduction in any medium, provided the original work is properly cited.

action on telomere maintenance, plays a major contribution in carcinogenesis and drug resistance. This enzyme is activated in almost 90% of cancers, including neuroblastoma (NBL).

Neuroblastoma is a malignant tumor of the peripheral sympathetic nervous system and the most common extracranial solid tumor in childhood [1, 2]. NBL is remarkably heterogeneous and displays a wide spectrum of differentiation stages from benign ganglioneuroma and well-differentiated tumors to undifferentiated malignant NBL. NBL is also a heterogeneous disease in terms of outcome and response to treatments: from spontaneous regression to resistance to all known treatments. In about 60% of the cases, NBL is diagnosed as a disseminated high-risk disease (stage 4), and most are diagnosed after 18 months of age. Genomic amplification of *MYCN* (V-Myc avian myelocytomatosis viral oncogene neuroblastoma-derived homolog) has been strongly associated with unfavorable patient outcome in approximately 20% of primary neuroblastoma tumors and approximately 40% of high-risk NBL. This alteration has thus been established as a robust marker for the definition of high-risk NBL. However, that *MYCN* amplification occurs only in 40% of high-risk NBL indicates that other genetic and/or epigenetic alterations play an important role in this disease. Array comparative genomic hybridizations have been widely employed to discover genome abnormalities and evaluate patient's risk. NBL displays several numerical and structural copy number variations such as the loss of 1p, 3p, 9p, 11q, and 14q, and the gain of 1q, 2p, and 17q, which identify high-risk subsets of NBL [3, 4]. That aggressive stage 4 neuroblastoma expressed high levels of telomerase activity, whereas favorable tumors had no or little telomerase expression and activity [5, 6], suggest an important role of this enzyme in the biology of neuroblastoma and its response to chemotherapy. NBL has a very low mutation frequency. The most two mutated genes are *ALK* (anaplastic lymphoma kinase) coding a tyrosine kinase, altered in about 7–8% of all primary tumors and 50% of familial NBL cases [7, 8], and *ATRX* (alpha thalassemia/mental retardation syndrome, X-linked) in about 10% of NBL and generally found in older patients.

Recently, the next-generation sequencing has shown that high-risk NBLs are characterized by defects that in common lead to the activation of telomere maintenance pathways supporting the idea that targeting these pathways will benefit to the patients [9, 10].

Many excellent recent reviews [11, 12] already exist on telomeres and telomerase in many aspects (structure and functions, regulation, and epigenetic control). This paper will therefore briefly review the recent knowledge on this topic, then, it will focus on the mechanisms of telomerase reactivation and telomere length maintenance in NBL, and discuss how these regulatory mechanisms can be targeted or "manipulated" for therapeutic purposes to modify cell fate and anticancer drug response in NBL.

2. Telomeres and telomerase

2.1. Telomeres

Every normal human somatic cell has a molecular clock for dividing, a process discovered by Leonard Hayflick, half a century ago, who observed that diploid cells in culture can divide only a limited number of times before stopping in a state known as the cellular senescence or the "Hayflick limit" [13]. In eukaryotic organisms, conventional DNA polymerases alone cannot fully replicate the ends of linear chromosomes, called telomeres. Therefore, telomere ends are progressively shortened after each cellular division [14, 15]. This leads to genomic instability and senescence or apoptosis.

Telomeres are specialized nucleoprotein structures made of 10–15 kb of short non-protein-coding repetitive 5′-TTAGGG-3′ DNA sequences. Telomeric DNA is mainly double-stranded, terminating in a single-stranded 3′ G-rich overhang of 150–200 nucleotides (nt) [16, 17]. These double-stranded repeats have one guanosine-rich strand (G-strand) copied by the lagging-strand replication, and one cytosine-rich strand (C-strand) synthesized by leading-strand replication. The telomeric DNAs are bound by shelterin protein complexes consisting of telomeric repeat factors 1 and 2 (TRF1 and TRF2), repressor/activator protein 1 (RAP1), TRF1- and TRF2-interacting nuclear protein 2 (TIN2), tripeptidyl-peptidase 1 (TPP1), and protection of telomeres 1 (POT1) [18, 19]. TRF1 and TRF2 bind to the double-stranded telomere DNA repeats, whereas POT1 binds to the single-stranded G-rich overhang. The three remaining proteins of the shelterin complex act as adaptors to mediate the interactions between the complex constituents: POT1 interacts with TPP1, a ternary complex of other proteins (TINT1/PTOP/PIP1), which interacts in turn with TIN2 that plays a key role in stabilizing the shelterin complex *via* its interaction with TPP1, TRF1, and TRF2. TPP1 also plays a major role in controlling the recruitment of the telomerase to the telomeres. RAP1 binds to TRF2 and acts as a mandatory element to the formation of the t-loop and the protection of the telomeres from the non-homologous end-joining (NHEJ) process. This process is dependent on the ataxia telangiectasia-mutated (ATM) kinase, the ataxia telangiectasia, and Rad3 (ATR) kinase, involved in the repair of the double-stranded and the single-stranded DNA breaks, respectively.

Due to the tandem organization of the G-rich telomeric DNA, the telomeres can form specialized four-stranded helical structures that involve Hoogsten-type base pairing between four guanines, named G-quadruplex (or G4) [20]. Alternatively, the G-strand overhang is also involved in the formation of the t-loop in which it invades the double-stranded region [21]. It has been hypothesized that those structures, which are not mutually exclusive, are able, by sequestering the 3′ end, to prevent the extension of the telomeres by telomerase.

Besides their role of capping chromosomes and protecting them from being recognized as DNA breaks [22], telomeres ensure proper chromosome segregation during mitosis [23] as well as transcriptional silencing of genes located close to them. Indeed, telomere shortening can alter gene expression by a process named telomere position effect (TPE) [24]. This process leads to the reversible silencing of genes near the telomere and thus is dependent on telomere length. In yeast, TPE can repress genes located up to 20 kb from the end [25, 26]. Recently, using a Hi-C (chromosome capture followed by high-throughput-sequencing) technique, three genes located at three different subtelomeric ends (1p, 6p, and 12p) were reported to have their expression altered with telomere length: *ISG15* (interferon-stimulated gene 15kD), *DSP* (Desmoplakin), and *C1S* (complement component 1s subcomplement). This phenomenon occurs through chromosomal looping between the loci of these genes and their respective telomere ends [27, 28]. Therefore, many loci may be regulated by telomere length.

This observation provides a new potential mechanism by which telomere shortening could contribute to the aging process and cancer development.

Two mechanisms of telomere maintenance have been identified in humans: the telomerase-mediated maintenance observed in 90% of cancers and, in the remaining 10%, the alternative lengthening of telomeres (ALT), which depends on homologous recombination [29, 30].

2.2. Telomerase: a ribonucleoprotein complex with multiple functions

Elizabeth Blackburn and her graduate student Carol Greider (2009 Nobel Prize in Physiology or Medicine) who worked on the ciliated protozoan *Tetrahymena thermophila* identified the enzyme responsible for the telomeric repeat synthesis [31]. This ribonucleoprotein (RNP) enzyme maintains telomere length by adding repetitive sequences to chromosome ends, slowing down telomere attrition [32].

Telomerase is an RNA-dependent DNA polymerase that plays a key role in carcinogenesis. By synthesizing telomeric DNA at the termini of chromosomes and stabilizing telomere lengths, it overcomes the senescence barrier due to the progressive telomere shortening associated with cell divisions [33]. Normal human somatic cells have very low or undetectable telomerase activity. By contrast, this activity has been detected in a wide range of human cancers (85–90%), in stem cells and adult germline tissues [34, 35]. By its action on telomeres, this enzyme confers to cancer cells their infinite cell proliferation potential and controls cell survival [36–38]. Telomerase is believed to be a significant target in cancer therapy since its upregulation appears to be a feature of malignant cells.

The human telomerase is a ribonucleoprotein enzyme (127 kDa) composed of at least two components, a catalytic subunit, telomerase reverse transcriptase (hTERT), and a template RNA component (hTR) (**Figure 1**).

hTR is a non-polyadenylated 451-nt long non-coding RNA containing eight conserved regions (CR1–CR8) that acts mainly as a template for the synthesis of the telomeric DNA. hTR binds hTERT *via* a template-pseudoknot domain (CR1/CR2) and a stem-loop domain (CR4/CR5) located in the middle of this RNA structure, which interacts with the DNA-binding domain of hTERT (**Figure 1**). hTERT protein functions as a dimer in the telomerase complex. Additional proteins are also required for a functional telomerase complex *in vivo*: small nucleolar RNPs, NHP2 (non-histone protein 2), NOP10 (nucleolar protein 10), GAR1, shelterin, and the ATPases Pontin and Reptin [39, 40]. The shelterin complex aids at the stabilization of the 3′ end at the telomeres. The appropriate stabilization of hTR and its proper interaction with hTERT involves the recruitment of dyskerin (DKC1), an RNA-binding protein, facilitated by the ATPases Reptin and Pontin [41]. The assembly of telomerase occurs in the nucleus in the Cajal bodies, and its localization at telomeres requires TCAB1 (Telomerase CAjal Body protein 1) and TPP1 proteins [42, 43].

Loss-of-function mutations of either *hTERT* or *hTR* are associated with pathologies such as aplastic anemia, pulmonary fibrosis, and dyskeratosis congenital, diseases characterized by stem cell depletion, deficiency in tissue regeneration, and tissue atrophy [44].

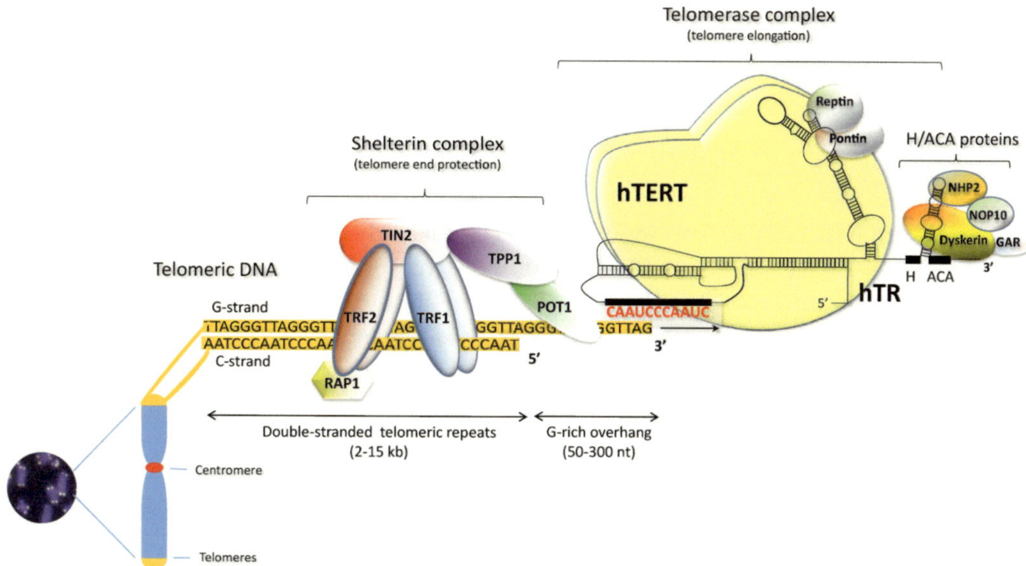

Figure 1. The human telomere and telomerase: the human telomerase is composed at least of telomerase reverse transcriptase (hTERT), telomerase RNA component (hTR), and accessory proteins that are members of the H/ACA small nucleolar ribonucleoprotein family: dyskerin; NHP2 (non-histone protein 2); NOP10 (nucleolar protein 10); GAR1 ribonucleoprotein.

Besides its canonical role, accumulated evidence indicates that telomerase elicits other functions in several essential cell-signaling pathways, including apoptosis, differentiation, DNA damage responses, and regulation of gene expression [45–50]. Even though these functions appear independent of telomerase activity, it is not excluded that some transient effect at telomeres can affect chromatin structure and gene expression. One example of these non-canonical functions of hTERT is the demonstration that hTERT binds NF-κB p65 subunit and regulates some of its target genes such as *IL (Interleukin)-6, IL-8, TNF (tumor necrosis factor) α*, and matrix metallo proteinases (*MMPs*) [51, 52]. In turn, NF-κB (nuclear factor κ-light-chain-enhancer of activated B cells) can activate the expression of hTERT by binding to its promoter indicating a feed-forward loop between telomerase and NF-κB [53]. hTERT protein can also function as a transcriptional modulator of the Wnt (wingless-related integration site)/β-catenin-signaling pathway [54]. Indeed, hTERT and β-catenin co-associate at the Wnt/β-catenin target gene promoters by forming a complex with the ATPase subunit of SWI/SNF (switch/sucrose non-fermentable) chromatin-remodeling complex, BRG1 (Brahma-related gene 1). Interestingly both wild-type and catalytically inactive hTERT led to the reactivation of Wnt/β-catenin target genes suggesting that this function is independent of its conventional function at telomeres. In turn, the Wnt/β-catenin pathway regulates the expression of hTERT in embryonic stem cells and in cancer cells through the recruitment of β-catenin to the promoter of *hTERT* indicating, in this case also, a positive feed-forward loop between telomerase and β-catenin [55]. Furthermore, functioning as an RNA-dependent RNA polymerase, hTERT has been implicated in the production of small-interfering (si) RNAs in a Dicer-dependent manner and thereby is involved in posttranscriptional gene silencing [56]. This activity of hTERT occurs through the interaction of hTERT protein with BRG1 and nucleostemin [57, 58]. For example, hTERT, through this activity, mediates the production of endogenous siRNAs using the RNA component of the mitochondrial RNA-processing endonuclease (RMRP) as a template.

Recently, it has been shown that BRG1 plays an essential role in maintaining the proliferation and viability of NBL cells. Interestingly, BRG1 is consistently upregulated in several NBL cell lines and in advanced stages of NBLs. Furthermore, high BRG1 levels have been correlated with poor patient outcome [59]. Therefore, BRG1 inhibition could be a possible new line of treatment for high-risk NBL patients. In view of these observations, the relationship between BRG1 and hTERT in NBL should be investigated.

2.3. Human hTERT regulation

Given the key role of telomerase in malignant transformation and tumor progression, great efforts have been deployed to unravel the mechanisms underlying telomerase activation.

2.3.1. hTERT gene and its promoter

The *hTERT* gene is 42-kb (kilobases) long with 16 exons [60] located in humans on the short arm of chromosome 5 (5p15.33) [61], more than 2 Mb away from telomeres. The reverse transcriptase domain is coded by exons 5–9. Differential splicing of *hTERT* mRNA has been demonstrated during embryonal development in various tissues. So far, 22 isoforms have been described resulting from alternative splicing [62, 63]; however, only the full-length isoform, which retains the reverse transcriptase activity, is able to elongate telomeres [64, 65]. Variants that lack the reverse transcriptase domain could affect telomerase activity by acting as competitive inhibitors as reported for the α-variant [66] or may have by themselves telomere-independent activities [62, 67, 68]. However, these experiments should be interpreted cautiously because they are based on overexpression conditions that are far beyond the physiological conditions.

Telomerase activity is generally well correlated with *hTERT* expression indicating that *hTERT* is a key regulator of this enzyme. *hTERT* gene is mostly regulated at the transcriptional level. This regulation is complex and includes multiple levels [69, 70].

The *hTERT* promoter does not have typical transcription-regulatory elements as TATA or CAAT boxes but is GC-rich. The core promoter harbors at least five GC boxes and two E-boxes (enhancer boxes with the canonical sequence of 5′-CACGTG-3′), which are sites for Sp1 (specificity protein 1), and c-Myc-binding, respectively, as well as multiple other transcription factor-binding sites involved in *hTERT* gene transcription: E-26 (ETS) family members, E2F, AP1 (activator protein 1), p53, p21, HIF (hypoxia-inducible factor), NF-kB, β-catenin, CTCF (CCCTC-binding factor), WT1 (Wilms′ tumor 1), and MZF2 (myeloid zinc finger 2) [71] (**Figure 2**).

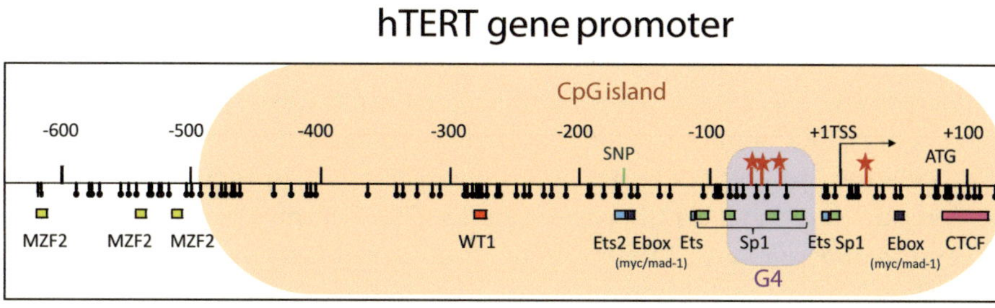

Figure 2. Schematic representation of the *hTERT* promoter: binding sites for various transcription factors are shown. The transcription start site (TSS, +1) and the translation start site (ATG, +78) are indicated. Stars indicate hotspot promoter mutations. The rs2853669 polymorphism (SNP) is shown in the ETS2-binding site. CTCF: CTCF factor-binding site; E-Box: Myc/Mad-family factor-binding site; Sp1: binding site for the SP1 transcription factor; ETS: ETS-domain site; WT1: binding site for the Wilms' tumor 1 transcription factor; MZF2: binding site for the myeloid zinc finger 2 transcription factor. Vertical tick marks with dark circles indicate the location of CpG dinucleotides. G4 indicates the localization of the G-quadruplex structure that can be adopted by *hTERT* promoter.

2.3.2. *Transcriptional regulators of hTERT*

The factors that bind *hTERT* promoter were characterized as transcriptional activators or transcriptional repressors or can play both roles depending on the cell type and the cellular context. Different factors can sometimes compete for binding to the same site or cooperate for binding to adjacent sites on *hTERT* promoter. Most of the studies concern the effect of transcription factors interacting with the core region of *hTERT* promoter, spanning from −180 bp (base pair) upstream to +1 bp downstream of the transcription start site. However, transcription factors interacting with a more distant region can also play an important role. Their action can be modulated by epigenetic modifications (see below). Therefore, the transcriptional level of *hTERT* results from a complex regulatory network of all these factors. These latter observations can explain the contradictory results that are reported in the literature. Given the complexity of *hTERT* regulation, it is difficult to integrate all the information. In addition, many factors indirectly regulate *hTERT* transcription through their interaction with other signaling pathways. All these processes ensure a tight and coordinated control of the *hTERT* gene in order to silence it in most human somatic adult cells. This control is lost in most malignant cells.

Recent articles have already reviewed exhaustively the roles of specific regulatory factors of *hTERT* [33, 71, 72]. Here, we have selected the most important ones, those whose binding has been demonstrated by *in vivo* assays, and also those that could be involved in the physiopathology of neuroblastomas.

2.3.2.1. *c-Myc/Max/Mad-1*

c-Myc and its dimerization partner Max (Myc-associated factor X) bind to regulatory elements called E-boxes and recruits histone acetyltransferases in order to activate the transcription of various genes, including *hTERT* [73]. c-Myc binds to two canonical E-box sequences

(5′-CACGTC-3′) found in the core promoter of *hTERT* (at −165 and +44 bp from the transcription start site). This binding leads to the upregulation of *hTERT* gene, and the increase in telomerase activity [74, 75]. However, c-Myc alone is not always sufficient to upregulate the expression of *hTERT* suggesting the requirement of additional factors. For example, the cooperation between Sp1 and c-Myc has been demonstrated to upregulate *hTERT* expression in human foreskin keratinocytes transduced by E6 [76]. Recently, it has been reported that c-Myc can exert a dual role on *hTERT* promoter. Indeed, besides its action as a transcriptional activator of *hTERT*, c-Myc can also maintain its promoter in a repressive state [77]. This latter action is independent of the two E-boxes.

Numerous factors thereby are able to indirectly upregulate *hTERT* expression through their action on c-Myc expression: transforming growth factor (TGF)-β/Smad signaling, estrogen, Aurora-A, Survivin, Leptin, mitogen-activated protein kinase (MAPK)/PI3K (phosphoinositol-3-kinase)-signaling pathway, MMP9, and Sirtuin 1 (SIRT1). Conversely, many factors are able to repress *hTERT* expression by counteracting the c-Myc expression or activity. The most important one is Mad-1 (Max dimerization protein 1), a potent antagonist of c-Myc, which acts as a direct competitor for dimerization with Max and binding on the E-boxes. Other factors are also known to act on c-Myc expression and/or inhibit its binding to *hTERT* promoter: breast cancer 1 (BRCA1), p27KIP21, HIF-1alpha, and so on.

Despite the strong evidence of the action of c-Myc as a transcriptional activator of *hTERT*, several studies reported the lack of correlation between c-Myc expression and hTERT mRNA levels [78, 79]. However, in these studies, the direct binding of c-Myc on *hTERT* promoter has not been investigated.

NBL cells generally do not express c-Myc but N-MYC, a protein belonging to the same family. c-Myc and N-MYC are encoded by different genes but have similar structures and domains. As c-Myc, N-MYC protein was shown to be recruited to the *hTERT* promoter and to activate it in NBL [80]. However, it is not known whether N-MYC can always functionally replace c-Myc in *hTERT* regulation. Moreover, hTERT has been shown to regulate c-Myc protein stability by interacting directly with c-Myc suggesting the existence of a feed-forward loop. In addition, in c-Myc-driven lymphoma, hTERT can also be recruited to c-Myc target promoters [81]. Such a crosstalk between hTERT and N-MYC protein has not been reported in NBL yet.

2.3.2.2. Specificity protein 1 (Sp1)

Sp1 is a transcription factor that binds to GC-box motifs in the promoter of *hTERT*. It activates *hTERT* gene expression in telomerase-positive cells but suppresses it in telomerase-negative one [82]. Sp1 may work in cooperation with c-Myc to upregulate *hTERT* expression. However, in cooperation with Sp3, another GC-box binding protein, Sp1 can also suppress the expression of *hTERT*.

It is important to note that this GC-rich region of *hTERT* promoter is able to form a tandem G-quadruplex structure [83]. The formation and stabilization of these structures that involves at least three of the five Sp1-binding sites could, therefore, interfere with *hTERT* transcriptional regulation.

2.3.2.3. *Nuclear factor κ-light-chain-enhancer of activated B cells (NF-kB)*

NF-kB is a transcription factor complex playing a role in telomerase expression and activity either directly through its binding on *hTERT* promoter or indirectly through the modulation of the expression of transcription factors known to affect *hTERT* expression. The binding site of NF-kB on *hTERT* promoter is located 600 bp upstream of the ATG translation start codon. However, recently, another pathway for the activation of *hTERT* by this complex has been proposed. This new mechanism involves a hotspot *hTERT* promoter mutation (see below).

2.3.2.4. *Upstream stimulatory factor (USF) proteins*

As c-Myc, USF proteins bind directly to E-box motifs on the core promoter of *hTERT*. They play both activating and repressing roles in the regulation of *hTERT* gene expression depending on the cell context.

2.3.2.5. *CCCTC-binding factor*

CTCF transcription factor binds at the beginning of exon 1 (+4 to +39 bp) and near the beginning of exon 2 (+422 to +440 bp) relative to the ATG in *hTERT* promoter. It is a repressor of hTERT transcription. CTCF is unable to bind to methylated DNA and therefore its binding is dependent on the degree of DNA methylation [84].

2.3.2.6. *Wilms, tumor protein 1*

WT1 is described as a repressor of *hTERT*. Its binding site lies from −358 to −349 bp on *hTERT* promoter [85]. However, similar to CTCF, the binding of WT1 is known to be methylation-sensitive. This observation was further supported by Azouz et al. whose experiments, in an acute promyelocytic leukemia (APL) cell model, showed that hypermethylation of a distal domain of *hTERT* promoter induced by retinoic treatment prevented WT1 binding and therefore, the subsequent *hTERT* gene repression [86]. A recent study reports an inverse correlation between *WT1* expression and *MYCN* amplification and expression. Moreover, a high expression of WT1 has been associated with a poor outcome only for patients showing non-*MYCN*-amplified tumors [87]. In a cohort of 67 primary NBL tumors, no significant correlation between WT1 and hTERT expression was found ($p = 0.056$), whereas, considering only stage 4 tumors ($n = 51$), there was a significant higher WT1 expression in patients with a low hTERT expression ($p = 0.033$).[1]

2.3.3. *hTERT promoter mutations*

Recently, hotspot promoter recurrent mutations were identified first in sporadic and familiar malignant melanoma [88, 89]. These mutations, which cause an adenine-to-cytosine (A>C) mutation or a cytosine-to-thymine (C>T) transition at chromosome 5: 1,295,161, 1,295,228, and

[1] E. Ségal-Bendirdjian et al., unpublished results.

1,295,250 (−57, −124, and −146 bp upstream of the ATG translation start codon), are named −57A>C (or A161C), −124C>T (or C228T), and −146C>T (or C250T), respectively. From there, the *hTERT* promoter mutations have been identified in various types of cancers with different frequencies [90]. The two main mutations, −124C>T and −146 C>T, have been suggested to be oncogenic drivers on the basis of experimental data showing that (1) their introduction into the *hTERT* promoter reporter could significantly enhance the promoter activity [91]; (2) the creation of these mutations by genome editing in *hTERT* promoter of human pluripotent stem cells is sufficient to inhibit the repression of *hTERT* gene transcription normally observed in wild-type *hTERT* promoter-bearing stem cells after induction of differentiation [92]; and (3) tumors carrying *hTERT* promoter mutations were frequently observed to express higher levels of *hTERT* mRNA and telomerase activity compared with those carrying a wild-type promoter. The frequency of the −124C>T mutation is generally higher than the frequency of the −146C>T mutations (80 vs. 20%). Other less common mutations were also detected in the *hTERT* promoter such as the CC>TT mutations at −124/−125 (Chr.5: 1,295,228–1,295,229) and −138/−139 (Chr.5: 1,295,242–1,295,243) positions. Note that these mutations occur in the G-rich region of the promoter known to form G-quadruplex structures [83]; therefore they can abrogate their negative effect on transcription by changing their stability and/or altering their recognition.

hTERT promoter mutation rates vary significantly from undetectable to 85% among studied human cancer types. The mutations occur most frequently in bladder, thyroid, hepatocellular cancers, malignant glioblastoma, and melanoma [93–96], while they are rarely present in hematological malignancies, prostate, gastrointestinal, breast, and lung cancers [90, 97, 98]. That a high frequency of *hTERT* promoter mutations was found in a multitude of advanced cancers suggests their key role in the reactivation of telomerase activity.

Mechanistically, −124C>T or −146C>T mutation generates an 11-base nucleotide stretch (5′-CCCCTTCCGGG-3′), which contains a consensus-binding site (GGAA in reverse complement) for ETS family transcription factors [99]. It was shown that the multimeric GA-binding protein (GABP), an ETS family transcription factor, was specifically recruited to the mutant rather than wild-type *hTERT* promoter in different cancer cells. This recruitment is associated with an enhanced enrichment of active chromatin leading to the opening of chromatin, an increased recruitment of PolII, and upregulation of *hTERT* expression and activity [91, 100]. This effect is further enhanced by the activation of the non-canonical NF-kB-signaling pathway. Indeed, the recruitment of the p52 subunit of NF-kB to the C250T site facilitates the stimulation of *hTERT* transcription.

Genome-wide association studies revealed the presence of single-nucleotide polymorphisms (SNPs) within the *hTERT* locus that were associated with increased risks in a variety of cancers. For example, rs2736100, located in intron 2, was associated with various types of cancer as glioma and colorectal cancer [101, 102]. Another SNP, rs2853669, found at *hTERT* promoter upstream of the first E-box, disrupts an ETS2-binding site [103, 104] and also hampers c-Myc binding to the adjacent E-box. The presence of this SNP can modify the effects of *hTERT* promoter mutations [105].

While *hTERT* promoter mutations have been identified in a broad range of cancers, not all cancers possess these mutations suggesting that other mechanisms contribute to hTERT reactivation.

2.3.4. *Epigenetic regulation of hTERT transcription*

The *hTERT* promoter is located in a 4-kb CpG island from −1800 to +2200 bp (relative to the TSS). Besides the involvement of transcription factors, epigenetic control and overall chromatin structure at *hTERT* promoter add another layer of hTERT regulation. It is well established that DNA methylation, histone acetylation, and methylation are also involved in the regulation of *hTERT* transcription even though the precise role and the molecular mechanisms are not well understood and even contradictory due to the different cellular models studied and the various methods used to analyze these epigenetic modifications.

Considering the methylation pattern categorized in different cell lines, it is possible to narrow the promoter to only two regions: one methylated, sometimes hypermethylated (from −650 to −200 bp from ATG) and one unmethylated or only slightly methylated (from −200 to +100 bp) [86, 106–110].

It is known that DNA methylation at gene promoter plays a major role in transcription factor binding. For example, hypomethylation at the *hTERT* core promoter may allow the binding of c-Myc to the E-boxes. Some reports, including ours, suggest that DNA methylation of *hTERT* promoter might have a key role in *hTERT* expression, but in a way opposite to what has been proposed so far. The hypothesis is that DNA methylation at *hTERT* promoter can contribute to prevent the binding of repressors and could account for high *hTERT* expression. This has been demonstrated for two transcription factors known to repress *hTERT*: CTCF whose binding site is located in exon 1 [71, 111, 112] and WT1 whose binding site is located in the distal promoter [86].

Besides DNA methylation, histones contribute to chromatin organization. Modifications can occur to their amino acid tails: methylation and acetylation are the most common. In general, methylation of histone 3 at its lysine 4 (H3K4) and hyperacetylation of histones are signs of hypo- or unmethylated DNA and active transcription gene. On the contrary, methylation of lysine 9 and 27 of histone 3 (H3K9 and H3K27, respectively) and hypoacetylation of histones are signs of hypermethylated DNA, so inactive transcription gene [110].

2.4. Human *TR* regulation

As *hTERT* is generally expressed only in telomerase-positive cells and its ectopic introduction alone can immortalize normal human cells, hTERT has been regarded as the limiting component of telomerase activity and much of the research has thus focused on the regulation of hTERT gene. However, even though *hTR* is ubiquitously expressed, evidence supports the notion that *hTR* can be also limiting for telomerase activity and telomere maintenance [113]. Indeed, the gene encoding *hTR*, a single-copy gene located on chromosome 3 at 3q26.3 [114], is highly regulated. A number of transcription-binding sites have been validated by either electrophoretic mobility gel gift assays, promoter reporters, and chromatin immunoprecipitation (ChIP) experiments, including Sp1, Sp3, and NF-Y [115, 116]. Furthermore, different signaling pathways have also been implicated in *hTR* transcription as JNK pathway.

3. Telomeres and telomerase in neuroblastoma

3.1. Telomerase as a biological marker and predictive factor in neuroblastoma

Several distinguishable groups in NBL have been identified based on their telomere biology and telomerase activation suggesting that telomerase expression may be one critical step in the development of neuroblastoma [5]. High telomerase activity allowing the maintenance of telomere length has been previously reported to correlate with advanced stages of the disease and with poor prognosis [5, 117–121]. By contrast, tumors without detectable telomerase activity showed favorable outcomes and some tumors regressed or matured [122]. This phenomenon of spontaneous regression led to propose a specific pattern of the metastatic disease called stage 4S. Children with stage 4S were restricted to infants aged less than 12 months at diagnosis, had generally small primary tumors with dissemination limited to the liver and skin and minimum bone marrow involvement [123]. The mechanisms involved in this regression remain to be elucidated. The expression of the alternate splice variants of *hTERT* could constitute a negative regulatory mechanism of telomerase at the posttranscriptional level and might account for the favorable evolution of these tumors [119, 124]. Therefore, full-length *hTERT* expression and telomerase activity, due to its strong correlation with the biological behavior of neuroblastoma tumors, may prove to be a good indicator of malignancy, in particular in 4S neuroblastoma. This may have consequences in the therapeutic strategies that can be adopted for these patients. As this form presents similar features as classic stage 4, it can be therefore treated as a high-risk group although in these cases, less therapeutic intensity could be given.

Several mechanisms have been proposed to explain the phenomenon of spontaneous regression. These include the neurotrophin receptor signaling when deprivation in nerve growth factor occurs, immune-mediated killing by anti-neural antibodies in patients, epigenetic regulation of gene expression through DNA methylation, histone modifications or chromatin remodeling, and finally telomere shortening and consequently apoptosis. Indeed, most of the tumor samples from 4S NBL have low telomerase activity or short telomeres [5]. This mechanism is further supported by Samy et al. who showed that a neuroblastoma cell line transfected by a dominant-negative form of human telomerase was more prone to apoptosis and had reduced tumorigenicity in a mouse xenograft model compared to untransfected neuroblastoma cells [125].

A correlation between *hTR* expression in primary NBLs, stage of disease, and survival [126, 127] has also been reported demonstrating a potential role for *hTR* as a biomarker even though most of the studies focused on *hTERT* expression. However, *hTR* expression does not always correlate with telomerase activity. This can be explained by the complexity of the different molecular mechanisms involved in telomerase regulation.

Even though the main role of telomerase is to maintain telomere length in tumors, non-canonical functions could also promote tumor growth and contribute to poor prognosis in primary NBLs (Wnt signaling, DNA repair, genomic instability, apoptosis, and escape from oncogene-induced senescence) [117].

Using a novel approach of three-dimensional (3D) telomere quantitative fluorescence *in situ* hybridization on 74 NBL tissue samples, a recent report demonstrates a possible classification of NBLs based on the level of telomere dysfunction, telomere length, and nuclear organization. Telomere dysfunctions were associated with unfavorable tumor characteristics, including *MYCN* amplification, and poor prognosis [128].

3.2. Potential mechanisms of hTERT activation and/or telomere maintenance mechanisms in neuroblastoma

The mechanisms by which telomerase activity is activated in high-stage NBL remain elusive. However, recent studies have shed some light on this important question. Although some controversies may remain, hTERT expression upregulation may occur through at least two pathways: *MYCN* amplification and genomic rearrangements around *hTERT*. Alternatively, ALT pathway can be activated in the absence of telomerase activation providing a mean for tumor cells to stabilize their telomeres as a necessary requirement for the immortalization and progression of the tumors.

3.2.1. MYCN amplification

MYCN amplification is the best characterized genetic marker and a powerful prognostic indicator of high-risk neuroblastoma [3]. *MYCN*-amplified tumors usually exhibit high telomerase activity and expression [118]. As developed earlier, c-Myc-binding sites are present on *hTERT* gene promoter and it is now well demonstrated that this factor, alone, or in cooperation with other transcription factors, determines the activity of *hTERT* promoter. N-MYC and c-Myc proteins are highly homologous. As c-Myc, N-MYC heterodimerizes with Max at consensus E-box sequences, therefore, *MYCN* overexpression could promote telomere stabilization through a transcriptional increase of *hTERT* gene expression associated with an increase in telomerase activity even though only one study reported such a direct interaction by ChIP in NBL [80]. An inverse correlation of *MYCN* and *c-Myc* expression was found in NBL subtypes [129]. As mentioned earlier, whether N-MYC protein can replace all c-Myc functions for *hTERT* regulation is still an unanswered question. Several lines of evidence suggest that MYC family members have separate physiological functions. The interplay between N-MYC and hTERT in NBL needs, thus, to be further investigated.

A recent study shows that *DKC1* gene promoter is targeted by both c-Myc and N-MYC and that high DKC1 expression is an independent prognostic indicator for adverse clinical outcome in NBL. *DKC1* gene encodes the RNA-binding protein dyskerin, a core component of the telomerase holoenzyme. This new function of DKC1 in NBL appears to be telomerase-independent [130].

3.2.2. hTERT promoter mutations

Although hotspot mutations in *hTERT* promoter driving telomerase activity are frequently described in neural crest-derived tumors such as melanoma [88, 89] and in a variety of other neuronal tumors including medulloblastoma and glioma [90, 131, 132], no *hTERT* promoter mutations have been detected in a large series (n = 131) of primary neuroblastoma [133], in line with previous studies performed on a smaller number of patients [90, 134]. However, these mutations were searched only in the core promoter of *hTERT*; it is not excluded that mutations may exist in more distant regulatory elements. The existence of a given SNP should also be searched.

3.2.3. hTERT gains

Chromosome 5p is often amplified in NBL, and focal *hTERT* gains were recently detected in several stage 4 primary NBLs. *hTERT* gains were more frequently detected in *MYCN* non-amplified cases, suggesting that *hTERT* gain performs a function similar to *MYCN* amplification [135, 136]. As N-MYC protein can bind and activate *hTERT* promoter, it is likely that *hTERT* gains are selected in order to increase hTERT expression in the absence of *MYCN* amplification.

3.2.4. hTERT rearrangements

Recent whole-genome sequencing of primary neuroblastoma, performed by two independent groups, discovered recurrent genomic rearrangements in a 70-kb region proximal to *hTERT* locus on the chromosome 5p15.33 [9, 10].

Indeed, in the first study [10], the authors were searching for structural alterations that might occur in high-risk NBL and, analyzing 56 tumors, they identified 4 locations exhibiting clustered breakpoints. These are related to *MYCN* amplifications, *ATRX* deletions, copy number gains of chromosome 17q, and rearrangements located at chromosome 5p15.33 proximal to *hTERT* gene. *hTERT* rearrangements occurred in 21% of tumors and included balanced translocations, copy number gains, high-level amplifications, and chromothripsis [137]. Chromothripsis corresponds to a massive and localized genome rearrangement [138], affecting high-risk tumors. Chromothripsis occurs in 2–3% of human cancers and, in a whole-genome-sequencing study, it occurs in 18% of high-risk NBL [137]. In an extended case series (n = 217), the authors showed that *hTERT* rearrangements are associated with a poor patient outcome and occur in mutually exclusive fashion with *MYCN* amplification and *ATRX* mutations (see below). They do not affect directly the *hTERT* gene or its promoter but they are all associated with an increase in *hTERT* transcription and telomerase activity as well as genes present in its vicinity (*SLC6A18* and *SLC6A19*) [139]. ChIP sequencing of *hTERT*-rearranged tumors indicated next to the breakpoints the presence of histone modifications known to mark active promoters (H3K4me3 and H3K27ac) and transcription elongation (H3K36me3), whereas in cells lacking *hTERT* alterations the repressive mark H3K27me3 was identified. Therefore, the structural rearrangement occurring at 5p15.33 results in a massive chromatin remodeling of this genomic region. The biological effect is the repositioning of regulatory elements very close to *hTERT* locus that could be responsible for the high induction of *hTERT* expression (up to 90 times that of normal cells) in these tumors.

In a similar whole-sequencing study [9] screening 108 NBLs, structural rearrangements of *hTERT* associated with hTERT overexpression were identified in 23% of cases. In *hTERT*-rearranged NBLs, a significant increase in telomere length has been demonstrated compared to non-rearranged NBLs. Both studies describe *hTERT* rearrangement as the second most frequent genetic defect in high-risk NBL after *MYCN* alteration. It is important to note that in those cases the promoter and coding regions of *hTERT* gene remain non-altered.

These results have been major advances in our understanding of NBL genetic and biology placing telomere biology at the core of this pathology.

3.2.5. Small nucleolar ribonucleoproteins (snoRNPs)

A recent study reported that the expression of proteins involved in the formation and stabilization of snoRNP complex (including DKC1, GAR1, and NHP2 proteins) is elevated in high-risk NBL and associated with poor prognosis. Furthermore, this study shows a positive correlation between DKC1 expression and telomerase activity. This increase is associated with an increase of *hTR* expression. Therefore, in NBL, upregulation of snoRNPs may contribute to telomere maintenance and stabilization [140].

3.2.6. ALT and neuroblastoma: ATRX (alpha thalassemia/mental retardation syndrome, X-linked) mutations

Telomere length does not necessarily correlate with telomerase activity [141]. Recently, it has been reported that some neuroblastomas (generally associated with unfavorable NBL in older children without *MYCN* amplification and regardless of telomerase activation status) preserve their telomere length in the absence of telomerase through telomere-binding proteins and alternative lengthening of telomeres, a process based on DNA repair/homologous recombination pathways [141–143]. ALT tumors represent 10–20% of NBL. These tumors have a very poor outcome. Phenotypically, ALT cells present long and heterogeneous telomere lengths [144], ALT-associated promyelocytic leukemia (PML) nuclear bodies [145], and abundant extra-chromosomal telomeric repeats [146]. A recent whole-genome-sequencing study identifies, in most ALT NBL cases, loss-of-function mutations in *ATRX* [137, 147, 148]. *ATRX* maps to the X chromosome and encodes a SWI/SNF chromatin-remodeling ATP-dependent helicase. ATRX regulates chromatin structure at both centromeric heterochromatin and telomeric regions [149]. In vitro analyses demonstrate its binding to GC-rich sequences and to G-quadruplexes [150]. Loss of ATRX functions may allow the destabilization of repressive heterochromatin at telomeres. NBLs with *ATRX* mutations show longer telomeres. *ATRX* mutations include in-frame deletions, missense, nonsense, and frameshift single-nucleotide variations. They are predominantly observed in adolescent and young adult patients (44% in patients older than 12 years, whereas no mutation was detected in infants <18 months of age [148]) and are frequently associated with chemo-resistance. ATRX protein establishes a functional interaction with DAXX (death domain-associated protein). At telomeres, ATRX and

DAXX proteins cooperate to deposit the histone H3 variants, H3.3, to maintain chromosome stability [151]. Loss of function of *ATRX/DAXX* is also associated with ALT activation [152] and poor overall survival among older patients. As mentioned earlier, *ATRX* mutations were mutually exclusive from *MYCN* amplification. However, how *ATRX* mutations lead to NBL progression is still an unanswered question.

3.2.7. ARID1A and ARID1B

Next-generation sequencing, genome-wide rearrangements analyses, and targeted analysis of specific genomic loci of 71 NBL patients identified mutations in chromatin-remodeling complexes encoded by *ARID1A/1B* (AT-rich interaction domain 1A/1B) genes in 11% of cases with decreased survival of patients [147]. Both proteins are subunits of the SWI/SNF transcriptional complex. They have emerged as tumor-suppressor genes and thereby when mutated can drive NBL tumorigenesis. However, additional studies will be required to elucidate the role of these proteins in the initiation or progression of NBL.

In conclusion, it is important to note that through either *MYCN* amplification, *hTERT* rearrangements, or *ATRX/DAXX* mutations, most high-risk NBLs have activated mechanisms, all of which are involved in the maintenance of telomere length and contribute to the tumor progression. This relationship highlights the major role of telomere/telomerase biology in NBL. These three mechanisms identify therefore distinct groups of NBL patients at very high risk with poor outcome [139]. That low-risk tumors lack such alterations support the notion that these kinds of tumors are more prone to spontaneously regress.

Altogether, these observations provide new important mechanisms that could be targeted in new therapeutic strategies to treat the most aggressive forms of neuroblastoma.

4. Telomerase, a target for cancer therapeutics

That, on one hand, both *MYCN* amplification and 5p15.33 rearrangement targeting *hTERT* locus lead to an increase in telomerase activity and subsequent telomere lengthening, and on the other hand ALT pathway is activated in tumors lacking *hTERT* or *MYCN* alterations indicate that the fate of high-risk NBL is largely dependent on telomerase/telomere biology. These new findings may help to improve tumor diagnostics and prognosis but also supports the development of novel therapeutic strategies targeting telomere/telomerase to treat the most aggressive form of this disease. Different molecules were shown to target telomerase by different mechanisms such as nucleoside analogs and reverse transcriptase inhibitors (zidovudine, stavudine, and tenofir), synthetic non-nucleoside inhibitors as BIBR1532 (2-[(E)-3 naphtalen-2-yl-but-2enoylamino]-benzoic acid), natural compounds (EGCG, MST-132), G-quadruplex stabilizers (telomestatin, BRACO-19), and molecular chaperone inhibitors affecting hTERT assembly (Hsp90 inhibitors). However, these compounds generally lack specificity and have adverse effects, and for now, no clinically validated drug targeting telomerase has been successfully developed. GRN163L (imetelstat), a phosphoramidate oligonucleotide targeting the template region of hTR, has undergone clinical trials by Geron Corporation (Menlo Park,

http://dx.doi.org/10.5772/intechopen.69567

CA, USA) [153–155]. However, the phase II study has been discontinued in breast cancers and non-small-cell lung carcinoma because no significant improvement in median progression-free survival was demonstrated. Moreover, hematological toxicity has been observed. However, these side effects have been used to propose this drug in hematological diseases. A phase II study evaluating the activity of imetelstat in patients with essential thrombocythemia or polycythemia vera is in progress. However, the actual mechanism of action of this molecule is still to be determined. For now, no clinical trials have been performed on NBL.

Regarding NBL, perhaps future attempts could be to target specifically N-MYC protein in patients who have NBL with *MYCN* amplification. However, the lack of specificity of the strategies targeting directly transcription factors is still a major concern. Bromodomain and extra terminal (BET) inhibitors, as JQ1 to specifically downregulate *MYCN* expression, are at the preclinical stage of evaluation [156]. Small molecules have been identified to inhibit c-Myc/Max interaction as well as decrease c-Myc protein levels and inhibit cell growth [157]. It has been shown that these molecules also interfere with N-MYC/Max interaction resulting in cell cycle arrest in *MYCN*-overexpressing NBL cell lines [158]. The consequences on hTERT expression have not been investigated yet.

The recent identification of *ATRX* mutations associated with their consequences on telomere structure in a specific group of high-risk NBL patients suggests that G-quadruplex stabilizers could be a potential therapeutic strategy to partially reverse the effects of *ATRX* mutations.

Telomerase expression was proposed as a selectively targetable mechanism for retinoids and specifically all *trans* retinoic acid (ATRA), an already clinically relevant drug used to stimulate differentiation of APL. Indeed, in a APL cellular model, it has been shown that retinoids can induce transcriptional repression of *hTERT* gene not only in differentiation of sensitive cells but also in cells resistant to ATRA-induced differentiation [159–161]. As the mechanism of *hTERT* repression occurs at the level of gene transcription, all the functions of telomerase can thus be targeted. Therefore, it is worth considering this antitelomerase property of retinoids in combination with more conventional therapies to target NBL. A recent study reporting the efficacy of a combination therapy, using retinoids and epigenetic modulators, in reducing NBL cell growth supports this idea [162].

5. Conclusions

Several potential chemotherapy strategies based on telomerase and telomere biology have been developed and explored by pharmaceutical and biotechnology companies [163]. However, in spite of ever-growing knowledge on telomere and telomerase biology, a number of questions remain to be answered as most of these numerous strategies are not yet clinically available because of a weak efficiency and/or a high toxicity. Therefore, to develop agents that will be effective, we need a sharper picture of how the enzyme functions and how we can manage to target specifically and destabilize telomeres in cancer cells. Epigenetic therapies aimed at counteracting the genetic alterations (mutations) are emerging alternatives against aggressive tumors.

Telomerase regulation is highly complex, involving the interplay between numerous biological and molecular processes. Despite the extensive studies that have been already done, a lot more is necessary to unravel the mechanisms underlying the switching off/on of *hTERT* gene during cell differentiation and cell transformation. However, progress in this direction is hampered by the absence of standardized methods to measure hTERT expression and telomerase activity and the lack of suitable tools in the study of telomere/telomerase biology.

First, telomerase repeated amplification protocol (TRAP) assay is a rather artificial assay to quantify telomerase activity; it is based on a quantitative real-time polymerase chain reaction (PCR) method that measures only the capacity of the telomerase reverse transcriptase to elongate artificial telomeric substrates without giving any measurement of the other functions of this protein. To date, no assay exists to evaluate the non-conventional functions of hTERT.

Second, *hTERT* expression is generally quantified using also a quantitative real-time PCR; however, in most cases it is not clearly known which *hTERT* isoform (full-length or specific splice variants) is detected. This would explain why, sometimes, comparison between telomerase activity and *hTERT* transcripts yielded contradictory results. Indeed, generally exhaustive measurements using different primer sets for the detection of various *hTERT* isoforms are not usually done. The detection and quantification of splice variants can be of interest for clinical outcome and prognosis. Moreover, further studies are also required to define precisely the functions of these variants.

Third, *hTR* is rarely quantified; however, it is also a limiting factor in telomere homeostasis.

Finally, due to the low expression of telomerase even in cancer cells, the detection of telomerase by western blot or fluorescence is puzzling. In addition, commercially available anti-hTERT antibodies are still a problem with specificity [164]. Because of these limitations, several published studies used overexpressed hTERT protein (generally tagged). However, the unusually high concentration of the protein due to the overexpression could alter the dynamic and the localization of the protein compared to the endogenous protein leading to misinterpretations.

Since the first paper published in 1995 [5], very few scientific advances have been done on a potential involvement of telomere/telomerase in NBL biology. However, the recent findings highlighting the role of telomere/telomerase biology in high-risk NBL will definitely impact the research in this pathology as well as in other cancers and help to develop new therapeutic strategies.

Acknowledgements

The work of the authors was supported by grants from the French National Institute of Health and Medical Research (INSERM), the National Center for Scientific Research (CNRS), the Ligue Nationale contre le Cancer, the Fondation de France (n° 201300038226), the French National Research Agency (ANR), Gefluc, Agence Universitaire de la Francophonie (AUF), Hubert Curien Partnership (PHC-CEDRE), and Ministère de l'Enseignement Supérieur et de la Recherche (MESR). Yann Blondin is acknowledged for his help in preparing **Figure 1**.

http://dx.doi.org/10.5772/intechopen.69567

Author details

Joëlle El Hajj[1,2,3], Delphine Garsuault[1,3], Claire Bouyer[1], Eric Nguyen[1], George Hilal[2] and Evelyne Ségal-Bendirdjian[1]*

*Address all correspondence to: evelyne.segal-bendirdjian@inserm.fr

1 INSERM UMR-S 1007, Cellular Homeostasis and Cancer, Paris Descartes University, Paris, France

2 Cancer and Metabolism Laboratory, Faculty of Medicine, Saint-Joseph University, Beirut, Lebanon

3 Paris-Sud University, Paris-Saclay University, Orsay, France

References

[1] Maris JM. Recent advances in neuroblastoma. The New England Journal of Medicine. 2010;**362**:2202-2211

[2] Brodeur GM. Neuroblastoma: Biological insights into a clinical enigma. Nature Reviews Cancer. 2003;**3**:203-216

[3] Brodeur GM, Seeger RC, Schwab M, Varmus HE, Bishop JM. Amplification of N-myc in untreated human neuroblastomas correlates with advanced disease stage. Science. 1984;**224**:1121-1124

[4] Cohn SL, Pearson AD, London WB, Monclair T, Ambros PF, Brodeur GM, et al. The International Neuroblastoma Risk Group (INRG) classification system: An INRG Task Force report. Journal of Clinical Oncology: Official Journal of the American Society of Clinical Oncology. 2009;**27**:289-297

[5] Hiyama E, Hiyama K, Yokoyama T, Matsuura Y, Piatyszek MA, Shay JW. Correlating telomerase activity levels with human neuroblastoma outcomes. Nature Medicine. 1995;**1**:249-255

[6] Poremba C, Hero B, Heine B, Scheel C, Schaefer KL, Christiansen H, et al. Telomerase is a strong indicator for assessing the proneness to progression in neuroblastomas. Medical and Pediatric Oncology. 2000;**35**:651-655

[7] Mosse YP, Laudenslager M, Longo L, Cole KA, Wood A, Attiyeh EF, et al. Identification of ALK as a major familial neuroblastoma predisposition gene. Nature. 2008;**455**:930-935

[8] Janoueix-Lerosey I, Lequin D, Brugieres L, Ribeiro A, de Pontual L, Combaret V, et al. Somatic and germline activating mutations of the ALK kinase receptor in neuroblastoma. Nature. 2008;**455**:967-970

[9] Valentijn LJ, Koster J, Zwijnenburg DA, Hasselt NE, van Sluis P, Volckmann R, et al. TERT rearrangements are frequent in neuroblastoma and identify aggressive tumors. Nature Genetics. 2015;**47**:1411-1414

[10] Peifer M, Hertwig F, Roels F, Dreidax D, Gartlgruber M, Menon R, et al. Telomerase activation by genomic rearrangements in high-risk neuroblastoma. Nature. 2015;**526**:700-704

[11] Wu RA, Upton HE, Vogan JM, Collins K. Telomerase mechanism of telomere synthesis. Annual Review of Biochemistry. 2017, in press

[12] Low KC, Tergaonkar V. Telomerase: Central regulator of all of the hallmarks of cancer. Trends in Biochemical Sciences. 2013;**38**:426-434

[13] Hayflick L. The limited in vitro lifetime of human diploid cell strains. Experimental Cell Research. 1965;**37**:614-636

[14] Blackburn EH. Switching and signaling at the telomere. Cell. 2001;**106**:661-673

[15] Levy MZ, Allsopp RC, Futcher AB, Greider CW, Harley CB. Telomere end-replication problem and cell aging. Journal of Molecular Biology. 1992;**225**:951-960

[16] Wright WE, Tesmer VM, Huffman KE, Levene SD, Shay JW. Normal human chromosomes have long G-rich telomeric overhangs at one end. Genes & Development. 1997;**11**:2801-2809

[17] Makarov VL, Hirose Y, Langmore JP. Long G tails at both ends of human chromosomes suggest a C strand degradation mechanism for telomere shortening. Cell. 1997;**88**:657-666

[18] de Lange T. How shelterin solves the telomere end-protection problem. Cold Spring Harbor Symposia on Quantitative Biology. 2010;**75**:167-177

[19] de Lange T. Shelterin: The protein complex that shapes and safeguards human telomeres. Genes & Development. 2005;**19**:2100-2110

[20] Sundquist WI, Klug A. Telomeric DNA dimerizes by formation of guanine tetrads between hairpin loops. Nature. 1989;**342**:825-829

[21] Stansel RM, de Lange T, Griffith JD. T-loop assembly in vitro involves binding of TRF2 near the 3′ telomeric overhang. The EMBO Journal. 2001;**20**:5532-5540

[22] Blackburn EH. Structure and function of telomeres. Nature. 1991;**350**:569-573

[23] Donate LE, Blasco MA. Telomeres in cancer and ageing. Philosophical Transactions of the Royal Society of London Series B, Biological Sciences. 2011;**366**:76-84

[24] Gottschling DE, Aparicio OM, Billington BL, Zakian VA. Position effect at *S. cerevisiae* telomeres: Reversible repression of Pol II transcription. Cell. 1990;**63**:751-762

[25] Stavenhagen JB, Zakian VA. Yeast telomeres exert a position effect on recombination between internal tracts of yeast telomeric DNA. Genes & Development. 1998;**12**:3044-3058

[26] Tham WH, Zakian VA. Transcriptional silencing at Saccharomyces telomeres: Implications for other organisms. Oncogene. 2002;**21**:512-521

[27] Kim W, Ludlow AT, Min J, Robin JD, Stadler G, Mender I, et al. Regulation of the human telomerase gene TERT by telomere position effect-over long distances (TPE-OLD): Implications for aging and cancer. PLoS Biology. 2016;**14**:e2000016

[28] Robin JD, Ludlow AT, Batten K, Magdinier F, Stadler G, Wagner KR, et al. Telomere position effect: Regulation of gene expression with progressive telomere shortening over long distances. Genes & Development. 2014;**28**:2464-2476

[29] Bryan TM, Englezou A, Dalla-Pozza L, Dunham MA, Reddel RR. Evidence for an alternative mechanism for maintaining telomere length in human tumors and tumor-derived cell lines. Nature Medicine. 1997;**3**:1271-1274

[30] Bryan TM, Marusic L, Bacchetti S, Namba M, Reddel RR. The telomere lengthening mechanism in telomerase-negative immortal human cells does not involve the telomerase RNA subunit. Human Molecular Genetics. 1997;**6**:921-926

[31] Greider CW, Blackburn EH. The telomere terminal transferase of tetrahymena is a ribonucleoprotein enzyme with two kinds of primer specificity. Cell. 1987;**51**:887-898

[32] Morin GB. The human telomere terminal transferase enzyme is a ribonucleoprotein that synthesizes TTAGGG repeats. Cell. 1989;**59**:521-529

[33] Ramlee MK, Wang J, Toh WX, Li S. Transcription regulation of the human telomerase reverse transcriptase (hTERT) gene. Genes. 2016;**7**:50

[34] Kim NW, Piatyszek MA, Prowse KR, Harley CB, West MD, Ho PL, et al. Specific association of human telomerase activity with immortal cells and cancer. Science. 1994;**266**: 2011-2015

[35] Armanios M, Greider CW. Telomerase and cancer stem cells. Cold Spring Harbor Symposia on Quantitative Biology. 2005;**70**:205-208

[36] Blackburn EH. Telomeres and telomerase: Their mechanisms of action and the effects of altering their functions. FEBS Letters. 2005;**579**:859-862

[37] Meyerson M, Counter CM, Eaton EN, Ellisen LW, Steiner P, Caddle SD, et al. hEST2, the putative human telomerase catalytic subunit gene, is up-regulated in tumor cells and during immortalization. Cell. 1997;**90**:785-795

[38] Feng J, Funk WD, Wang SS, Weinrich SL, Avilion AA, Chiu CP, et al. The RNA component of human telomerase. Science. 1995;**269**:1236-1241

[39] Podlevsky JD, Chen JJ. It all comes together at the ends: Telomerase structure, function, and biogenesis. Mutation Research. 2012;**730**:3-11

[40] Venteicher AS, Meng Z, Mason PJ, Veenstra TD, Artandi SE. Identification of ATPases pontin and reptin as telomerase components essential for holoenzyme assembly. Cell. 2008;**132**:945-957

[41] Mitchell JR, Wood E, Collins K. A telomerase component is defective in the human disease dyskeratosis congenita. Nature. 1999;**402**:551-555

[42] Venteicher AS, Abreu EB, Meng Z, McCann KE, Terns RM, Veenstra TD, et al. A human telomerase holoenzyme protein required for Cajal body localization and telomere synthesis. Science. 2009;**323**:644-648

[43] Venteicher AS, Artandi SE. TCAB1: Driving telomerase to Cajal bodies. Cell Cycle. 2009;**8**:1329-1331

[44] Dokal I. Dyskeratosis congenita. Hematology American Society of Hematology Education Program. 2011;**2011**:480-486

[45] Cong Y, Shay JW. Actions of human telomerase beyond telomeres. Cell Research. 2008; **18**:725-732

[46] Smith LL, Coller HA, Roberts JM. Telomerase modulates expression of growth-controlling genes and enhances cell proliferation. Nature Cell Biology. 2003;**5**:474-479

[47] Dudognon C, Pendino F, Hillion J, Saumet A, Lanotte M, Segal-Bendirdjian E. Death receptor signaling regulatory function for telomerase: hTERT abolishes TRAIL-induced apoptosis, independently of telomere maintenance. Oncogene. 2004;**23**:7469-7474

[48] Lee J, Sung YH, Cheong C, Choi YS, Jeon HK, Sun W, et al. TERT promotes cellular and organismal survival independently of telomerase activity. Oncogene. 2008;**27**:3754-3760

[49] Bollmann FM. The many faces of telomerase: Emerging extratelomeric effects. Bioessays. 2008;**30**:728-732

[50] Park JI, Venteicher AS, Hong JY, Choi J, Jun S, Shkreli M, et al. Telomerase modulates Wnt signalling by association with target gene chromatin. Nature. 2009;**460**:66-72

[51] Ding D, Zhou J, Wang M, Cong YS. Implications of telomere-independent activities of telomerase reverse transcriptase in human cancer. The FEBS Journal. 2013;**280**:3205-3211

[52] Ghosh A, Saginc G, Leow SC, Khattar E, Shin EM, Yan TD, et al. Telomerase directly regulates NF-kappaB-dependent transcription. Nature Cell Biology. 2012;**14**:1270-1281

[53] Yin L, Hubbard AK, Giardina C. NF-kappa B regulates transcription of the mouse telomerase catalytic subunit. The Journal of Biological Chemistry. 2000;**275**:36671-36675

[54] Listerman I, Gazzaniga FS, Blackburn EH. An investigation of the effects of the core protein telomerase reverse transcriptase on Wnt signaling in breast cancer cells. Molecular and Cell Biology. 2014;**34**:280-289

[55] Hoffmeyer K, Raggioli A, Rudloff S, Anton R, Hierholzer A, Del Valle I, et al. Wnt/beta-catenin signaling regulates telomerase in stem cells and cancer cells. Science. 2012;**336**:1549-1554

[56] Maida Y, Yasukawa M, Furuuchi M, Lassmann T, Possemato R, Okamato N, et al. An RNA-dependent RNA polymerase formed by TERT and the RMRP RNA. Nature. 2009;**461**:230-235

[57] Maida Y, Yasukawa M, Okamoto N, Ohka S, Kinoshita K, Totoki Y, et al. Involvement of telomerase reverse transcriptase in heterochromatin maintenance. Molecular and Cell Biology. 2014;**34**:1576-1593

[58] Okamoto N, Yasukawa M, Nguyen C, Kasim V, Maida Y, Possemato R, et al. Maintenance of tumor initiating cells of defined genetic composition by nucleostemin. Proceedings of the National Academy of Sciences of the United States of America. 2011;**108**:20388-20393

[59] Jubierre L, Soriano A, Planells-Ferrer L, Paris-Coderch L, Tenbaum SP, Romero OA, et al. BRG1/SMARCA4 is essential for neuroblastoma cell viability through modulation of cell death and survival pathways. Oncogene. 2016;**35**:5179-5190

[60] Cong YS, Wen J, Bacchetti S. The human telomerase catalytic subunit hTERT: Organization of the gene and characterization of the promoter. Human Molecular Genetics. 1999;**8**: 137-142

[61] Bryce LA, Morrison N, Hoare SF, Muir S, Keith WN. Mapping of the gene for the human telomerase reverse transcriptase, hTERT, to chromosome 5p15.33 by fluorescence in situ hybridization. Neoplasia. 2000;**2**:197-201

[62] Hrdlickova R, Nehyba J, Bose HR, Jr. Alternatively spliced telomerase reverse transcriptase variants lacking telomerase activity stimulate cell proliferation. Molecular and Cell Biology. 2012;**32**:4283-4296

[63] Kilian A, Bowtell DD, Abud HE, Hime GR, Venter DJ, Keese PK, et al. Isolation of a candidate human telomerase catalytic subunit gene, which reveals complex splicing patterns in different cell types. Human Molecular Genetics. 1997;**6**:2011-2019

[64] Saeboe-Larssen S, Fossberg E, Gaudernack G. Characterization of novel alternative splicing sites in human telomerase reverse transcriptase (hTERT): Analysis of expression and mutual correlation in mRNA isoforms from normal and tumour tissues. BMC Molecular Biology. 2006;**7**:26

[65] Wong MS, Wright WE, Shay JW. Alternative splicing regulation of telomerase: A new paradigm? Trends in Genetics: TIG. 2014;**30**:430-438

[66] Colgin LM, Wilkinson C, Englezou A, Kilian A, Robinson MO, Reddel RR. The hTERTalpha splice variant is a dominant negative inhibitor of telomerase activity. Neoplasia. 2000;**2**:426-432

[67] Listerman I, Sun J, Gazzaniga FS, Lukas JL, Blackburn EH. The major reverse transcriptase-incompetent splice variant of the human telomerase protein inhibits telomerase activity but protects from apoptosis. Cancer Research. 2013;**73**:2817-2828

[68] Mukherjee S, Firpo EJ, Wang Y, Roberts JM. Separation of telomerase functions by reverse genetics. Proceedings of the National Academy of Sciences of the United States of America. 2011;**108**:E1363-E1371

[69] Wick M, Zubov D, Hagen G. Genomic organization and promoter characterization of the gene encoding the human telomerase reverse transcriptase (hTERT). Gene. 1999;**232**:97-106

[70] Takakura M, Kyo S, Kanaya T, Hirano H, Takeda J, Yutsudo M, et al. Cloning of human telomerase catalytic subunit (hTERT) gene promoter and identification of proximal core promoter sequences essential for transcriptional activation in immortalized and cancer cells. Cancer Research. 1999;**59**:551-557

[71] Kyo S, Takakura M, Fujiwara T, Inoue M. Understanding and exploiting hTERT promoter regulation for diagnosis and treatment of human cancers. Cancer Science. 2008; **99**:1528-1538

[72] Daniel M, Peek GW, Tollefsbol TO. Regulation of the human catalytic subunit of telomerase (hTERT). Gene. 2012;**498**:135-146

[73] Khattar E, Tergaonkar V. Transcriptional regulation of telomerase reverse transcriptase (TERT) by MYC. Frontiers in Cell and Developmental Biology. 2017;**5**:1

[74] Wu KJ, Grandori C, Amacker M, Simon-Vermot N, Polack A, Lingner J, et al. Direct activation of TERT transcription by c-MYC. Nature Genetics. 1999;**21**:220-224

[75] Xu D, Popov N, Hou M, Wang Q, Bjorkholm M, Gruber A, et al. Switch from Myc/Max to Mad1/Max binding and decrease in histone acetylation at the telomerase reverse transcriptase promoter during differentiation of HL60 cells. Proceedings of the National Academy of Sciences of the United States of America. 2001;**98**:3826-3831

[76] Oh ST, Kyo S, Laimins LA. Telomerase activation by human papillomavirus type 16 E6 protein: Induction of human telomerase reverse transcriptase expression through Myc and GC-rich Sp1 binding sites. Journal of Virology. 2001;**75**:5559-5566

[77] Zhao Y, Cheng D, Wang S, Zhu J. Dual roles of c-Myc in the regulation of hTERT gene. Nucleic Acids Research. 2014;**42**:10385-10398

[78] Kirkpatrick KL, Newbold RF, Mokbel K. There is no correlation between c-Myc mRNA expression and telomerase activity in human breast cancer. International Seminars in Surgical Oncology. 2004;**1**:2

[79] Elkak AE, Meligonis G, Salhab M, Mitchell B, Blake JRS, Newbold M, et al. hTERT protein expression is independent of clinicopathological parameters and c-Myc protein expression in human breast cancer. Journal of Carcinogenesis. 2005;**4**:17

[80] Mac SM, D'Cunha CA, Farnham PJ. Direct recruitment of N-myc to target gene promoters. Molecular Carcinogenesis. 2000;**29**:76-86

[81] Koh CM, Khattar E, Leow SC, Liu CY, Muller J, Ang WX, et al. Telomerase regulates MYC-driven oncogenesis independent of its reverse transcriptase activity. The Journal of Clinical Investigation. 2015;**125**:2109-122

[82] Kyo S, Takakura M, Taira T, Kanaya T, Itoh H, Yutsudo M, et al. Sp1 cooperates with c-Myc to activate transcription of the human telomerase reverse transcriptase gene (hTERT). Nucleic Acids Research. 2000;**28**:669-677

[83] Palumbo SL, Ebbinghaus SW, Hurley LH. Formation of a unique end-to-end stacked pair of G-quadruplexes in the hTERT core promoter with implications for inhibition of telomerase by G-quadruplex-interactive ligands. Journal of the American Chemical Society. 2009;**131**:10878-10891

[84] Renaud S, Loukinov D, Bosman FT, Lobanenkov V, Benhattar J. CTCF binds the proximal exonic region of hTERT and inhibits its transcription. Nucleic Acids Research. 2005;**33**:6850-6860

[85] Sitaram RT, Degerman S, Ljungberg B, Andersson E, Oji Y, Sugiyama H, et al. Wilms' tumour 1 can suppress hTERT gene expression and telomerase activity in clear cell renal cell carcinoma via multiple pathways. British Journal of Cancer. 2010;**103**:1255-1262

[86] Azouz A, Wu YL, Hillion J, Tarkanyi I, Karniguian A, Aradi J, et al. Epigenetic plasticity of hTERT gene promoter determines retinoid capacity to repress telomerase in maturation-resistant acute promyelocytic leukemia cells. Leukemia. 2010;**24**:613-622

[87] Masserot C, Liu Q, Nguyen E, Gattolliat CH, Valteau-Couanet D, Benard J, et al. WT1 expression is inversely correlated with MYCN amplification or expression and associated with poor survival in non-MYCN-amplified neuroblastoma. Molecular Oncology. 2016;**10**:240-252

[88] Huang FW, Hodis E, Xu MJ, Kryukov GV, Chin L, Garraway LA. Highly recurrent TERT promoter mutations in human melanoma. Science. 2013;**339**:957-959

[89] Horn S, Figl A, Rachakonda PS, Fischer C, Sucker A, Gast A, et al. TERT promoter mutations in familial and sporadic melanoma. Science. 2013;**339**:959-961

[90] Killela PJ, Reitman ZJ, Jiao Y, Bettegowda C, Agrawal N, Diaz LA, Jr., et al. TERT promoter mutations occur frequently in gliomas and a subset of tumors derived from cells with low rates of self-renewal. Proceedings of the National Academy of Sciences of the United States of America. 2013;**110**:6021-6026

[91] Bell RJ, Rube HT, Kreig A, Mancini A, Fouse SD, Nagarajan RP, et al. Cancer. The transcription factor GABP selectively binds and activates the mutant TERT promoter in cancer. Science. 2015;**348**:1036-1039

[92] Chiba K, Johnson JZ, Vogan JM, Wagner T, Boyle JM, Hockemeyer D. Cancer-associated TERT promoter mutations abrogate telomerase silencing. Elife. 2015;**4**

[93] Liu T, Wang N, Cao J, Sofiadis A, Dinets A, Zedenius J, et al. The age- and shorter telomere-dependent TERT promoter mutation in follicular thyroid cell-derived carcinomas. Oncogene. 2014;**33**:4978-4984

[94] Nault JC, Mallet M, Pilati C, Calderaro J, Bioulac-Sage P, Laurent C, et al. High frequency of telomerase reverse-transcriptase promoter somatic mutations in hepatocellular carcinoma and preneoplastic lesions. Nature Communications. 2013;**4**:2218

[95] Wang K, Liu T, Liu L, Liu J, Liu C, Wang C, et al. TERT promoter mutations in renal cell carcinomas and upper tract urothelial carcinomas. Oncotarget. 2014;**5**:1829-1836

[96] Wang N, Liu T, Sofiadis A, Juhlin CC, Zedenius J, Hoog A, et al. TERT promoter mutation as an early genetic event activating telomerase in follicular thyroid adenoma (FTA) and atypical FTA. Cancer. 2014;**120**:2965-2979

[97] Liu T, Liang X, Bjorkholm M, Jia J, Xu D. The absence of TERT promoter mutations in primary gastric cancer. Gene. 2014;**540**:266-267

[98] Stoehr R, Taubert H, Zinnall U, Giedl J, Gaisa NT, Burger M, et al. Frequency of TERT promoter mutations in prostate cancer. Pathobiology: Journal of Immunopathology, Molecular and Cellular Biology. 2015;**82**:53-57

[99] Li Y, Zhou QL, Sun W, Chandrasekharan P, Cheng HS, Ying Z, et al. Non-canonical NF-kappaB signalling and ETS1/2 cooperatively drive C250T mutant TERT promoter activation. Nature Cell Biology. 2015;**17**:1327-1338

[100] Stern JL, Theodorescu D, Vogelstein B, Papadopoulos N, Cech TR. Mutation of the TERT promoter, switch to active chromatin, and monoallelic TERT expression in multiple cancers. Genes & Development. 2015;**29**:2219-2224

[101] Zhou P, Wei L, Xia X, Shao N, Qian X, Yang Y. Association between telomerase reverse transcriptase rs2736100 polymorphism and risk of glioma. The Journal of Surgical Research. 2014;**191**:156-160

[102] Kinnersley B, Migliorini G, Broderick P, Whiffin N, Dobbins SE, Casey G, et al. The TERT variant rs2736100 is associated with colorectal cancer risk. British Journal of Cancer. 2012;**107**:1001-1008

[103] Hsu CP, Hsu NY, Lee LW, Ko JL. Ets2 binding site single nucleotide polymorphism at the hTERT gene promoter--effect on telomerase expression and telomere length maintenance in non-small cell lung cancer. European Journal of Cancer. 2006;**42**:1466-1474

[104] Shen N, Lu Y, Wang X, Peng J, Zhu Y, Cheng L. Association between rs2853669 in TERT gene and the risk and prognosis of human cancer: A systematic review and meta-analysis. Oncotarget. 2017; in press

[105] Batista R, Cruvinel-Carloni A, Vinagre J, Peixoto J, Catarino TA, Campanella NC, et al. The prognostic impact of TERT promoter mutations in glioblastomas is modified by the rs2853669 single nucleotide polymorphism. International Journal of Cancer. 2016;**139**:414-423

[106] Zinn RL, Pruitt K, Eguchi S, Baylin SB, Herman JG. hTERT is expressed in cancer cell lines despite promoter DNA methylation by preservation of unmethylated DNA and active chromatin around the transcription start site. Cancer Research. 2007;**67**: 194-201

[107] Guilleret I, Benhattar J. Unusual distribution of DNA methylation within the hTERT CpG island in tissues and cell lines. Biochemical and Biophysical Research Communications. 2004;**325**:1037-1043

[108] Guilleret I, Benhattar J. Demethylation of the human telomerase catalytic subunit (hTERT) gene promoter reduced hTERT expression and telomerase activity and shortened telomeres. Experimental Cell Research. 2003;**289**:326-334

[109] Zhao X, Tian X, Kajigaya S, Cantilena CR, Strickland S, Savani BN, et al. Epigenetic landscape of the TERT promoter: A potential biomarker for high risk AML/MDS. British Journal of Haematology. 2016;**175**:427-439

[110] Lewis KA, Tollefsbol TO. Regulation of the telomerase reverse transcriptase subunit through epigenetic mechanisms. Frontiers in Genetics. 2016;**7**:83

[111] Renaud S, Loukinov D, Abdullaev Z, Guilleret I, Bosman FT, Lobanenkov V, et al. Dual role of DNA methylation inside and outside of CTCF-binding regions in the transcriptional regulation of the telomerase hTERT gene. Nucleic Acids Research. 2007;**35**:7372-7388

[112] Richardson RM, Nguyen B, Holt SE, Broaddus WC, Fillmore HL. Ectopic telomerase expression inhibits neuronal differentiation of NT2 neural progenitor cells. Neuroscience Letters. 2007;**421**:168-172

[113] Cairney CJ, Keith WN. Telomerase redefined: Integrated regulation of hTR and hTERT for telomere maintenance and telomerase activity. Biochimie. 2008;**90**:13-23

[114] Soder AI, Hoare SF, Muire S, Balmain A, Parkinson EK, Keith WN. Mapping of the gene for the mouse telomerase RNA component, Terc, to chromosome 3 by fluorescence in situ hybridization and mouse chromosome painting. Genomics. 1997;**41**:293-294

[115] Zhao JQ, Hoare SF, McFarlane R, Muir S, Parkinson EK, Black DM, et al. Cloning and characterization of human and mouse telomerase RNA gene promoter sequences. Oncogene. 1998;**16**:1345-1350

[116] Zhao J, Bilsland A, Hoare SF, Keith WN. Involvement of NF-Y and Sp1 binding sequences in basal transcription of the human telomerase RNA gene. FEBS Letters. 2003;**536**:111-119

[117] Coco S, Theissen J, Scaruffi P, Stigliani S, Moretti S, Oberthuer A, et al. Age-dependent accumulation of genomic aberrations and deregulation of cell cycle and telomerase genes in metastatic neuroblastoma. International Journal of Cancer. 2012;**131**:1591-1600

[118] Hiyama E, Hiyama K, Ohtsu K, Yamaoka H, Ichikawa T, Shay JW, et al. Telomerase activity in neuroblastoma: Is it a prognostic indicator of clinical behaviour? European Journal of Cancer. 1997;**33**:1932-1936

[119] Krams M, Hero B, Berthold F, Parwaresch R, Harms D, Rudolph P. Full-length telomerase reverse transcriptase messenger RNA is an independent prognostic factor in neuroblastoma. The American Journal of Pathology. 2003;**162**:1019-1026

[120] Streutker CJ, Thorner P, Fabricius N, Weitzman S, Zielenska M. Telomerase activity as a prognostic factor in neuroblastomas. Pediatric and Developmental Pathology: The Official Journal of the Society for Pediatric Pathology and the Paediatric Pathology Society. 2001;**4**:62-67

[121] Ohali A, Avigad S, Ash S, Goshen Y, Luria D, Feinmesser M, et al. Telomere length is a prognostic factor in neuroblastoma. Cancer. 2006;**107**:1391-1399

[122] Poremba C, Willenbring H, Hero B, Christiansen H, Schafer KL, Brinkschmidt C, et al. Telomerase activity distinguishes between neuroblastomas with good and poor prognosis. Annals of Oncology: Official Journal of the European Society for Medical Oncology. 1999;**10**:715-721

[123] Taggart DR, London WB, Schmidt ML, DuBois SG, Monclair TF, Nakagawara A, et al. Prognostic value of the stage 4S metastatic pattern and tumor biology in patients with metastatic neuroblastoma diagnosed between birth and 18 months of age. Journal of Clinical Oncology: Official Journal of the American Society of Clinical Oncology. 2011;**29**:4358-4364

[124] Krams M, Claviez A, Heidorn K, Krupp G, Parwaresch R, Harms D, et al. Regulation of telomerase activity by alternate splicing of human telomerase reverse transcriptase mRNA in a subset of neuroblastomas. The American Journal of Pathology. 2001;**159**:1925-1932

[125] Samy M, Gattolliat CH, Pendino F, Hillion J, Nguyen E, Bombard S, et al. Loss of the malignant phenotype of human neuroblastoma cells by a catalytically inactive dominant-negative hTERT mutant. Molecular Cancer Therapeutics. 2012;**11**:2384-2393

[126] Reynolds CP, Zuo JJ, Kim NW, Wang H, Lukens JN, Matthay KK, et al. Telomerase expression in primary neuroblastomas. European Journal of Cancer. 1997;**33**:1929-1931

[127] Choi LM, Kim NW, Zuo JJ, Gerbing R, Stram D, Lukens JN, et al. Telomerase activity by TRAP assay and telomerase RNA (hTR) expression are predictive of outcome in neuroblastoma. Medical and Pediatric Oncology. 2000;**35**:647-650

[128] Kuzyk A, Gartner J, Mai S. Identification of neuroblastoma subgroups based on three-dimensional telomere organization. Translational Oncology. 2016;**9**:348-356

[129] Westermann F, Muth D, Benner A, Bauer T, Henrich KO, Oberthuer A, et al. Distinct transcriptional MYCN/c-MYC activities are associated with spontaneous regression or malignant progression in neuroblastomas. Genome Biology. 2008;**9**:R150

[130] O'Brien R, Tran SL, Maritz MF, Liu B, Kong CF, Purgato S, et al. MYC-driven neuroblastomas are addicted to a telomerase-independent function of dyskerin. Cancer Research. 2016;**76**:3604-3617

[131] Remke M, Ramaswamy V, Peacock J, Shih DJ, Koelsche C, Northcott PA, et al. TERT promoter mutations are highly recurrent in SHH subgroup medulloblastoma. Acta Neuropathologica. 2013;**126**:917-929

[132] Koelsche C, Sahm F, Capper D, Reuss D, Sturm D, Jones DT, et al. Distribution of TERT promoter mutations in pediatric and adult tumors of the nervous system. Acta Neuropathologica. 2013;**126**:907-915

[133] Lindner S, Bachmann HS, Odersky A, Schaefers S, Klein-Hitpass L, Hero B, et al. Absence of telomerase reverse transcriptase promoter mutations in neuroblastoma. Biomedical Reports. 2015;**3**:443-446

[134] Papathomas TG, Oudijk L, Zwarthoff EC, Post E, Duijkers FA, van Noesel MM, et al. Telomerase reverse transcriptase promoter mutations in tumors originating from the adrenal gland and extra-adrenal paraganglia. Endocrine-Related Cancer. 2014;**21**: 653-661

[135] Kumps C, Fieuw A, Mestdagh P, Menten B, Lefever S, Pattyn F, et al. Focal DNA copy number changes in neuroblastoma target MYCN regulated genes. PLoS One. 2013;**8**:e52321

[136] Cobrinik D, Ostrovnaya I, Hassimi M, Tickoo SK, Cheung IY, Cheung NK. Recurrent pre-existing and acquired DNA copy number alterations, including focal TERT gains,

in neuroblastoma central nervous system metastases. Genes, Chromosomes & Cancer. 2013;**52**:1150-1166

[137] Molenaar JJ, Koster J, Zwijnenburg DA, van Sluis P, Valentijn LJ, van der Ploeg I, et al. Sequencing of neuroblastoma identifies chromothripsis and defects in neuritogenesis genes. Nature. 2012;**483**:589-593

[138] Stephens PJ, Greenman CD, Fu B, Yang F, Bignell GR, Mudie LJ, et al. Massive genomic rearrangement acquired in a single catastrophic event during cancer development. Cell. 2011;**144**:27-40

[139] Kawashima M, Kojima M, Ueda Y, Kurihara S, Hiyama E. Telomere biology including TERT rearrangements in neuroblastoma: A useful indicator for surgical treatments. Journal of Pediatric Surgery. 2016;**51**:2080-2085

[140] von Stedingk K, Koster J, Piqueras M, Noguera R, Navarro S, Pahlman S, et al. snoRNPs regulate telomerase activity in neuroblastoma and are associated with poor prognosis. Translational Oncology. 2013;**6**:447-457

[141] Onitake Y, Hiyama E, Kamei N, Yamaoka H, Sueda T, Hiyama K. Telomere biology in neuroblastoma: Telomere binding proteins and alternative strengthening of telomeres. Journal of Pediatric Surgery. 2009;**44**:2258-2266

[142] Kurihara S, Hiyama E, Onitake Y, Yamaoka E, Hiyama K. Clinical features of ATRX or DAXX mutated neuroblastoma. Journal of Pediatric Surgery. 2014;**49**:1835-1838

[143] Lundberg G, Sehic D, Lansberg JK, Ora I, Frigyesi A, Castel V, et al. Alternative lengthening of telomeres--an enhanced chromosomal instability in aggressive non-MYCN amplified and telomere elongated neuroblastomas. Genes, Chromosomes & Cancer. 2011;**50**:250-262

[144] Henson JD, Neumann AA, Yeager TR, Reddel RR. Alternative lengthening of telomeres in mammalian cells. Oncogene. 2002;**21**:598-610

[145] Yeager TR, Neumann AA, Englezou A, Huschtscha LI, Noble JR, Reddel RR. Telomerase-negative immortalized human cells contain a novel type of promyelocytic leukemia (PML) body. Cancer Research. 1999;**59**:4175-4179

[146] Nabetani A, Ishikawa F. Alternative lengthening of telomeres pathway: Recombination-mediated telomere maintenance mechanism in human cells. Journal of Biochemistry. 2011;**149**:5-14

[147] Sausen M, Leary RJ, Jones S, Wu J, Reynolds CP, Liu X, et al. Integrated genomic analyses identify ARID1A and ARID1B alterations in the childhood cancer neuroblastoma. Nature Genetics. 2013;**45**:12-17

[148] Cheung NK, Zhang J, Lu C, Parker M, Bahrami A, Tickoo SK, et al. Association of age at diagnosis and genetic mutations in patients with neuroblastoma. Journal of the American Medical Association. 2012;**307**:1062-1071

[149] Clynes D, Higgs DR, Gibbons RJ. The chromatin remodeller ATRX: A repeat offender in human disease. Trends in Biochemical Sciences. 2013;**38**:461-466

[150] Law MJ, Lower KM, Voon HP, Hughes JR, Garrick D, Viprakasit V, et al. ATR-X syndrome protein targets tandem repeats and influences allele-specific expression in a size-dependent manner. Cell. 2010;**143**:367-378

[151] Lewis PW, Elsaesser SJ, Noh KM, Stadler SC, Allis CD. Daxx is an H3.3-specific histone chaperone and cooperates with ATRX in replication-independent chromatin assembly at telomeres. Proceedings of the National Academy of Sciences of the United States of America. 2010;**107**:14075-14080

[152] Heaphy CM, de Wilde RF, Jiao Y, Klein AP, Edil BH, Shi C, et al. Altered telomeres in tumors with ATRX and DAXX mutations. Science. 2011;**333**:425

[153] Akiyama M, Hideshima T, Shammas MA, Hayashi T, Hamasaki M, Tai YT, et al. Effects of oligonucleotide N3'-->P5' thio-phosphoramidate (GRN163) targeting telomerase RNA in human multiple myeloma cells. Cancer Research. 2003;**63**:6187-6194

[154] Shammas MA, Koley H, Bertheau RC, Neri P, Fulciniti M, Tassone P, et al. Telomerase inhibitor GRN163L inhibits myeloma cell growth in vitro and in vivo. Leukemia. 2008;**22**:1410-1418

[155] Asai A, Oshima Y, Yamamoto Y, Uochi TA, Kusaka H, Akinaga S, et al. A novel telomerase template antagonist (GRN163) as a potential anticancer agent. Cancer Research. 2003;**63**:3931-3939

[156] Puissant A, Frumm SM, Alexe G, Bassil CF, Qi J, Chanthery YH, et al. Targeting MYCN in neuroblastoma by BET bromodomain inhibition. Cancer Discovery. 2013;**3**:308-323

[157] Yin X, Giap C, Lazo JS, Prochownik EV. Low molecular weight inhibitors of Myc-Max interaction and function. Oncogene. 2003;**22**:6151-6159

[158] Muller I, Larsson K, Frenzel A, Oliynyk G, Zirath H, Prochownik EV, et al. Targeting of the MYCN protein with small molecule c-MYC inhibitors. PLoS One. 2014;**9**:e97285

[159] Tarkanyi I, Dudognon C, Hillion J, Pendino F, Lanotte M, Aradi J, et al. Retinoid/arsenic combination therapy of promyelocytic leukemia: Induction of telomerase-dependent cell death. Leukemia. 2005;**19**:1806-1811

[160] Pendino F, Dudognon C, Delhommeau F, Sahraoui T, Flexor M, Bennaceur-Griscelli A, et al. Retinoic acid receptor alpha and retinoid-X receptor-specific agonists synergistically target telomerase expression and induce tumor cell death. Oncogene. 2003;**22**: 9142-9150

[161] Pendino F, Flexor M, Delhommeau F, Buet D, Lanotte M, Segal-Bendirdjian E. Retinoids down-regulate telomerase and telomere length in a pathway distinct from leukemia cell differentiation. Proceedings of the National Academy of Sciences of the United States of America. 2001;**98**:6662-6667

[162] Almeida VR, Vieira IA, Buendia M, Brunetto AT, Gregianin LJ, Brunetto AL, et al. Combined treatments with a retinoid receptor agonist and epigenetic modulators in human neuroblastoma cells. Molecular Neurobiology. 2016; in press

[163] Pendino F, Tarkanyi I, Dudognon C, Hillion J, Lanotte M, Aradi J, et al. Telomeres and telomerase: Pharmacological targets for new anticancer strategies? Current Cancer Drug Targets. 2006;**6**:147-180

[164] Wu YL, Dudognon C, Nguyen E, Hillion J, Pendino F, Tarkanyi I, et al. Immunodetection of human telomerase reverse-transcriptase (hTERT) re-appraised: Nucleolin and telomerase cross paths. Journal of Cell Science. 2006;**119**:2797-2806

Chapter 7

Epigenetic Approaches in Neuroblastoma Disease Pathogenesis

Francesca Felicia Caputi, Sanzio Candeletti and Patrizia Romualdi

Additional information is available at the end of the chapter

http://dx.doi.org/10.5772/intechopen.69566

Abstract

Neuroblastoma is an embryonal extracranial solid tumor originating from undifferentiated neural crest cell and it is the most common among children. Neuroblastoma is highly heterogeneous, and on these bases different outcomes are observed across the subtypes. Its clinical impact (~13% of all pediatric cancer mortality) has made this aggressive malignancy the focus of a considerable translational research effort. New insights into tumor biology are leading to the development of novel therapeutic approaches, which include small-molecule inhibitors as well as epigenetic approaches, noncoding-RNA, and cell-based immunologic therapies. Recently, chromatin immunoprecipitation with high-throughput sequencing and RNA-sequencing studies have demonstrated that epigenetic changes contribute to the aggressive pathophysiology of pediatric neuroblastoma disease. Epigenetic abnormalities are feature of human cancer cells and the epigenetic alterations may be the key toward tumorigenesis. In particular, the increase of deacetylation has been involved in epigenetically mediated tumor-suppressor gene silencing. In addition, several studies evaluated the 5-methylcytosine (5 mC) distribution patterns, which distinguish cancer cells from normal cells, and how CpG methylation contributes to the oncogenic phenotype.

In particular, histone changes and DNA methylation are fundamental biological processes representing versatile candidates for pharmacological manipulation with important therapeutic advantages.

Keywords: neuroblastoma, epigenetics, histone marks, DNA methylation, proteasome inhibitors

1. Introduction

Neuroblastoma is an embryonal extracranial solid tumor originating from undifferentiated neural crest cell and it is the most common among children. Neuroblastomas are highly

INTECH
open science | open minds

© 2017 The Author(s). Licensee InTech. This chapter is distributed under the terms of the Creative Commons Attribution License (http://creativecommons.org/licenses/by/3.0), which permits unrestricted use, distribution, and reproduction in any medium, provided the original work is properly cited.

heterogeneous, and on these bases different outcomes are observed across the subtypes from the spontaneous regression, asymptomatic tumors, as well as metastasized tumors to rapid progression and resistance to therapy. Its clinical impact (~13% of all pediatric cancer mortality) has made this aggressive malignancy the focus of a considerable translational research effort. Recent literature suggests that alterations in gene transcription programs drive disease-specific gene expression, thus highlighting the significance of transcription as a major mechanism for driving tumor growth and neoplastic transformation. In this chapter, the sophisticated language of the epigenetic code emerges as promising target for cancer therapy. It is generally accepted that epigenetic abnormalities are feature of human cancer cells and that epigenetic alterations may be the key toward tumorigenesis. Briefly, in eukaryotic nuclei, DNA is wrapped around an octameric histone (H) unit, which is composed of H2A, H2B, H3, and H4. This basic structure known as a nucleosome is repeated along the double-stranded DNA, with a fifth type of histone (the linker histone H1) bridging together consecutive nucleosomes (**Figure 1**). Based on the level of compaction, we can distinguish two main forms of chromatin: the euchromatin is the transcriptionally active form characterized by permissive marks such as the acetylation of different lysine residues; the heterochromatin is the transcriptionally silent configuration and contains repressive epigenetic marks [1]. These forms differ biochemically with respect to the presence of specific markers at the histone tails (see **Figure 2**) and to the binding of structural proteins.

Gene transcription in eukaryotic utilizes multiple mechanisms and it is mainly regulated by four families of the ATP-dependent chromatin-remodeling complexes (switching defective/sucrose non-fermenting = SWI/SNF; imitation-switch = ISWI; Mi-2/nucleosome remodeling and histone deacetylation = Mi-2/NuRD; inositol 80 = INO80), named "remodelers" [3–6]. A growing body

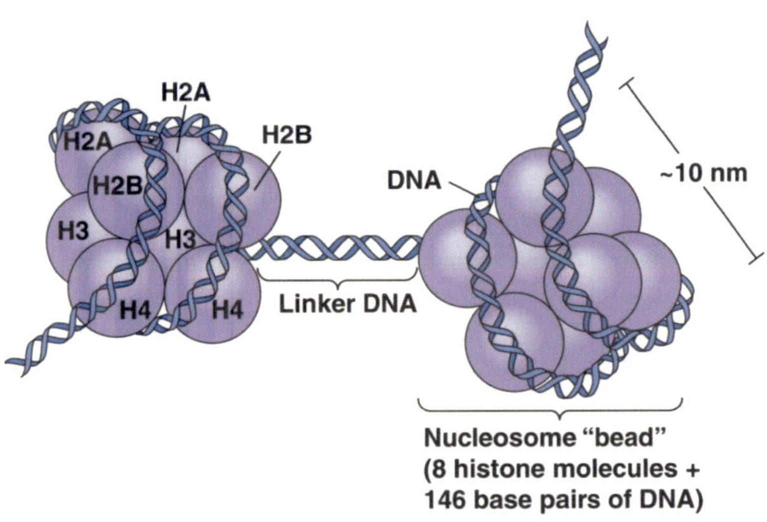

Figure 1. Schematic representation of the nucleosome. The nucleosome core is composed of a histone octamer [(H2A-H2B)×2, (H3-H4)×2]. The DNA double helix is wrapped around (~1.7 times) the histone octamer. With nuclease digestion, 146 bps of DNA are tightly associated with the nucleosome but ~200 bps of DNA in total are associated with the nucleosome [2].

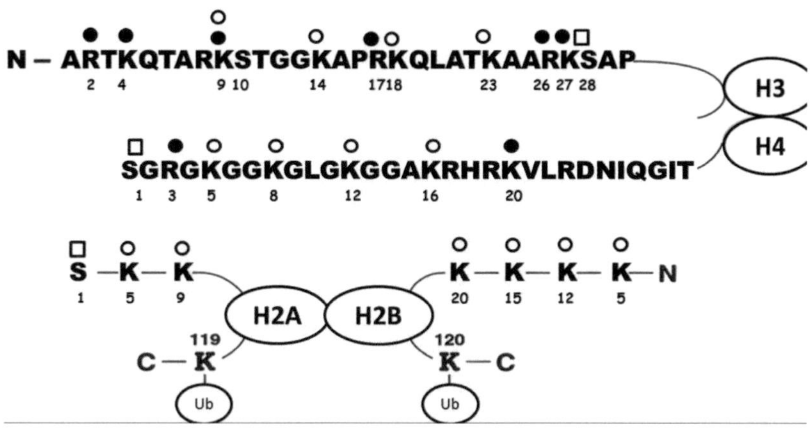

Figure 2. All histones are subject to post-transcriptional modifications (PTMs) which mainly occur on the histone tails. The main PTMs are depicted in this figure: acetylation (○), methylation (●), phosphorylation (□) and ubiquitination (Ub). The number under each amino acid [K = lysine (Lys), R = arginine (Arg) and S = serine (Ser)] represents its position in the sequence (Adapted from Zhang and Reinberg, 2001) [16]. In addition, the position K4, K9, K27, K36 and K79 can be mono-/di-/ or trimethylated.

of evidence suggests that the dysregulation of chromatin remodelers such as activating mutation, homozygous deletion, epigenetic silencing, and overexpression has a crucial role in cancer development and in its progression [7–10]. Advances in genomic technologies have allowed a better understanding of genomic signatures underlying human cancer.

1.1. Histone modifications

Histone tails are subject to different post-translational modifications (PTMs), including acetylation, methylation, and phosphorylation. The best characterized chromatin PTM is the histone acetylation, which results from a dynamic balance of the activity of two enzymatic families: histone acetyl-transferases (HATs) and histone deacetylases (HDACs) [11, 12]. Alterations in the balance of these enzyme activities lead to a disruption of cellular integrity and are frequently observed in different tumors. In particular, the increase of deacetylation has been involved in epigenetically mediated tumor-suppressor gene silencing; thus, HDACs represent a promising class of anticancer drug targets [13] (**Figure 2**).

Methylation of histone proteins is generally found on arginine and lysine residues. Three different forms of methylation have been observed on the lysine residues (mono-, di-, and trimethylation), whereas arginine can be mono-methylated and symmetrically or asymmetrically di-methylated; these modifications play different functions in gene transcription [14] (**Figure 2**). In fact, methylation of histones can either increase or decrease gene transcription, depending on which amino acids on the histones are methylated, and how many methyl groups are attached.

For example, trimethylation of lysine 4 on histone H3 (H3K4me3) is abundant at active gene promoter, whereas trimethylation of lysine 9 on histone H3 (H3K9me3) is associated with transcriptionally repressed gene promoters [15]. Histone methylation process is catalyzed by three distinct families of methyltransferase enzymes namely the SET-domain containing protein family, the non-SET domain protein family, and the protein arginine methyltransferase family 1 (PRMT1) [17]. Changes in histone methylation status take part in various physiological and pathological processes, including cancer.

1.2. DNA methylation

The understanding of DNA methylation contribution to cancer-specific alterations and the exact consequences of these mutations, in the key steps of tumorigenesis, will represent a useful tool in epigenetics therapy. In mammals, DNA methylation occurs predominantly at cytosine in CpG islands, and their methylation acts as a relatively stable gene-silencing mechanism. Over the last 40 years, several studies evaluated the 5-methylcytosine (5 mC) distribution patterns, which distinguish cancer cells from normal cells, and how CpG methylation contributes to the oncogenic phenotype.

DNA methylation is regulated by a family of DNA methyltransferases (DNMTs) which catalyze the transfer of methyl groups from S-adenosyl-L-methionine to the 5′ position of cytosine bases in the CpG dinucleotide. DNMT3A and DNMT3B establish new DNA methylation patterns early in development [19].

During replication, the original DNA methylation pattern is mainly maintained by DNMT1 activity, which prefers hemi-methylated DNA over non-methylated DNA as a substrate [20] and it is therefore responsible for the maintenance of methylation patterns during cell division, with some participation by DNMT3A and DNMT3B [21]. DNMT1, DNMT3A, and DNMT3B are often overexpressed in various cancers and they may contribute to the abnormal hypermethylation [18, 22].

In this view, it is interesting to note that the global DNA hypomethylation [18–20], the abnormal hypermethylation in promoter CpG islands [23–25] and the exact mutagenesis of sequences containing 5 mC [26, 27] may occur simultaneously suggesting that altered homeostasis of epigenetic mechanisms is central to the evolution of human cancer and plays an active role in increasing chromosomal fragility.

2. Epigenetics landscape in mammalian development

Notwithstanding the neuroblastoma, tumorigenesis arise from the disrupted development of neural crest precursors, no single genetic or epigenetic mutation has been found after the DNA and RNA sequencing of over 1000 cases [28]. Recently, chromatin immunoprecipitation with high-throughput-sequencing and RNA-sequencing studies have demonstrated specific epigenetic patterns which distinguish neuroectoderm, neural crest, and more mature neural states, since a cardinal property of neural stem cells (NSCs) is their ability to adopt multiple fates upon differentiation [29]. Fascinating studies focused their attention on the epigenome as indicator of cell fate, and numerous observations highlight significant alterations within chromatin structure during mammalian development [30, 31]. In this frame, the developmental epigenetic regulation is the most deeply documented in the embryonic stem cell (ESC) research. Even though many promoters of developmental genes in ESCs contain permissive as well as repressive epigenetic marks, they are transcriptionally silent and maintained in a transcriptionally silent state until differentiation [32]. Analogously, the NSCs differentiation is a unidirectional process tightly regulated to ensure the acquisition of specific neuronal phenotypes [33]. A novel chromatin modification pattern known as "bivalent domains" may explain these processes. Mainly, genes that are active in cells throughout development originally have active promoters which are characterized by the presence of the bivalent histone modification pattern consisting of H3K4me3 (permissive mark), trimethylation of lysine (K) 27 on histone H3 (H3K27me3, repressive mark), and a lack of DNA methylation. Genes enriched for K27me3 in ESC include those involved in early embryonic development, organogenesis, and cell fate decisions. In fact, genes that become transcriptionally active lose much of their polycomb-mediated repressive H3K27 methylation, conversely those that become silenced lose their H3K4 methylation or increases the polycomb-mediated repressive chromatin mark [32, 34]. However, recent works suggest that the loss of H3K27me3 is not sufficient to lead the increased transcription of all genes.

In the same direction, it has been shown that during the differentiation of ESC-derived NSCs, to immature GABAergic interneurons, all non-GABAergic promoters maintain the H3K27me3 repressive monovalency mark, whereas GABAergic promoters maintain the H3K4me3 mark (permissive monovalency) [29].

However, little is still known about the overall genomic distribution of K4 rather than K27 methylation in ESCs; the hypothesis is that bivalent domains consist of large regions of K27 methylation which hid smaller regions of K4 methylation. This bivalence condition is usually lost during ESC differentiation and in the differentiated cells [32].

Besides histone modification, the DNA methylation is equally essential for mammalian development and it is also linked to tumorigenesis [35, 36]. Unlike bivalent domains, cytosine methylation provides a methylated genome which can self-protect from environment changes due to the ability to repress specific promoters [37]. Among the three active DNA cytosine methyltransferases, identified in human and mouse [38, 39], the DNMT1 is responsible for copying the parental-strand methylation pattern onto the daughter strand after each round of DNA replication; DNMT3A and DNMT3B are strongly expressed in ESCs where they are essential for the de novo methylation and in maintaining methylation patterns [36, 40]. In 2003, it has been reported that the inactivation of both DNMT3A and DNMT3B results in progressive loss of methylation in various repeats and single-copy genes in ESCs. Moreover, the introduction of DNMT isoforms into highly demethylated mutant ESCs showed that the DNMT3A, DNMT3A2, and DNMT3B1 restore genomic methylation patterns, whereas DNMT1 and DNMT3B3 failed to restore DNA methylation patterns due to their inability to catalyze de novo methylation *in vivo* [41].

3. Novel therapeutic approaches in neuroblastoma

3.1. Epigenetic therapy

Since neuroblastoma is a complex disease, driven by multiple genetic and epigenetic alterations, it is subject of intensive ongoing genomic research. In particular, during tumor initiation and progression the epigenome goes through multiple alterations. Promoter hypermethylation of tumor-suppressor genes [42], together with promoter methylation of several DNA repair genes and histone modifications [43], is commonly observed in cancer cells. Neuroblastoma is frequently associated with numerous genetic alterations and in this regard it has been reported that the restored expression of the zinc-finger transcription factor castor (human castor gene: CASZ1) inhibits cell proliferation *in vitro* and decreases tumor growth *in vivo* [44]. In addition, the expression of CASZ1 appears significantly decreased in aggressive phenotype of patients with unfavorable prognoses [45], thus indicating CASZ1 as a tumor-suppressor gene in neuroblastoma tumor. However, the absence of consistent CpG methylation of CASZ1 in neuroblastoma excludes a gene-silencing mechanism due to DNA methylation [46]; on the contrary, it seems that trichostatin A, a histone deacetylase inhibitors, induces CASZ1 expression in neuroblastoma cells [46], suggesting an epigenetic mechanism mainly dependent on histone regulation. In addition, histone modifications may affect the recruitment of transcription factors and of other components of the transcription machinery, thereby contributing to aberrant gene expression [21]; notably, altered histone modifications have been found in neuroblastoma tumors and have been correlated to tumor aggressiveness [45, 47]. Despite this evidence, the epigenetic changes, which contribute to the aggressive pathophysiology of neuroblastoma, are still poorly known. In this frame, preclinical studies have demonstrated that the DNA methylation appears to play a role in angiogenesis inhibitor thrombospondin-1 (TSP-1) regulation [48]. Neuroblastoma growth might be closely related to angiogenesis, since the angiogenesis inhibitors downregulation has been observed in highly malignant neuroblastoma cells and the administration of antiangiogenesis agents successfully inhibits neuroblastoma growth *in vivo* [49, 50]. In this regard, Yang and colleagues tested the efficacy of 5-Aza-dC (a demethylating agent) to restore the TSP-1 transcription in the TSP-1-negative neuroblastoma cell lines confirming that the silencing of this gene was triggered by a methylation process (**Figure 3**) [48]. Therefore, demethylating agents may be effective candidates for neuroblastoma-affected children.

Because epigenetic changes caused by DNA methylation are critical for the initiation and for the cancer progression, it has been also demonstrated that aberrant splicing of DNMTs is frequently exhibited in cancer cells [22, 51]. Notably, it has been suggested that high levels of truncated DNMT3B7 isoform alter DNA methylation and might be related to embryonic development and a less aggressive clinical neuroblastoma phenotype [52]. To test this hypothesis, Ostler and colleagues forced the expression of DNMT3B7 isoform in neuroblastoma cells to evaluate its effects on DNA methylation, tumor growth, and angiogenesis. They observed an increase of global DNA methylation, the decrease of aggressive neuroblastoma growth, and the suppression of angiogenesis, respectively, consistent with a nonmalignant phenotype [52].

3.2. Combined therapy with proteasome inhibitor

The presence of cancer stem cell population in the neuroblastoma increases the migratory properties of cancer cells, and this is a major concern in cancer therapeutics since the relapse of tumor and resistance to therapy are due to the self-renewing cancer cells [53, 54]. Doxorubicin (Dox), a Food and Drug Administration (FDA)-approved chemotherapeutic agent widely used in numerous cancer type, would benefit neuroblastoma patients and lead to better outcomes [55].

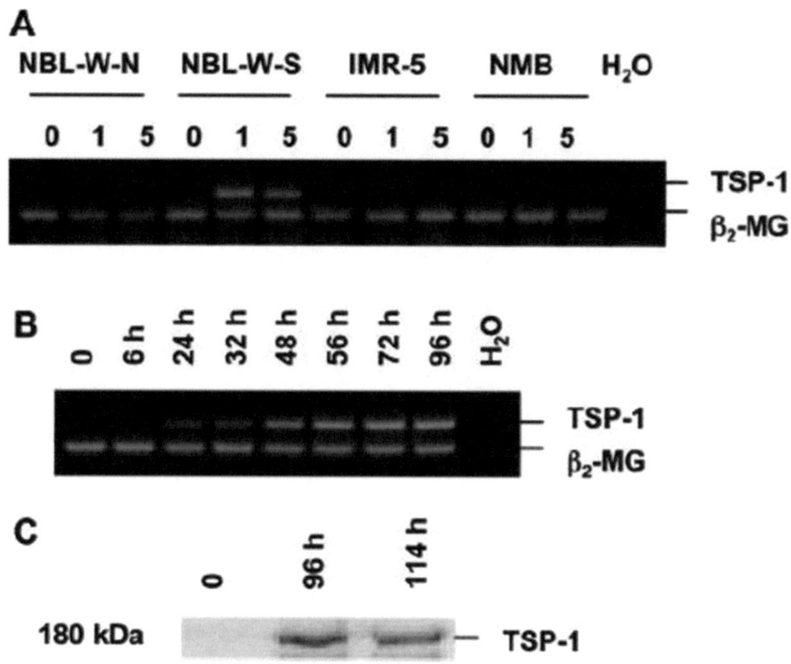

Figure 3. Reinstatement of TSP-1 after treatment with 5-Aza-dC. (A) TSP-1 gene expression levels were detected by RT-PCR analysis in NBL-W-S cells treated with vehicle or 1 or 5 μM of 5-Aza-dC for 60h; (B) time-dependent re-expression of TSP-1 following exposure to exposed to 1 μM of 5-Aza-dC; (C) Western blot analysis of TSP-1 expression after treatment with 5-Aza-dC (image from Yang et al., 2003) [48].

However, Dox induces nuclear factor-κB (NF-κB) activation which is believed to contribute to the development of chemoresistance [56]; thus, a viable option in cancer therapy could be the inhibition of NF-κB activation to overcome the chemoresistance. Among various biological systems exploited to obtain therapeutic benefits, the ubiquitin-proteasome system has been associated with tumor cell survival [57]. Notably, pharmacological inhibition of proteasome activity by small-molecule inhibitors shows anti-tumor efficacy in various cancer types [57]; proteasome activity has been also reported to be involved in NF-κB activation by promoting the degradation of its inhibitor IκBα [58].

Therefore, in order to improve therapeutic outcomes, the ability of Ixazomib to suppress neuroblastoma cell proliferation and to induce cell apoptosis has been recently reported. Ixazomib is a selective second-generation proteasome inhibitor able to enhance the Dox cytotoxicity (**Figure 4**) and capable to inhibit Dox-induced NF-κB activation [59]. Li and colleagues demonstrated the anti-tumor efficacy of Ixazomib in combination with Dox corroborating the hypothesis that combination therapies of proteasome inhibitors and chemotherapeutic agents will achieve better outcomes in neuroblastoma therapy. Similar results were also obtained using another second-generation proteasome inhibitor, the Carfilzomib [60] indicating the relevance of proteasome machinery in the therapeutic strategy for treating neuroblastoma patients.

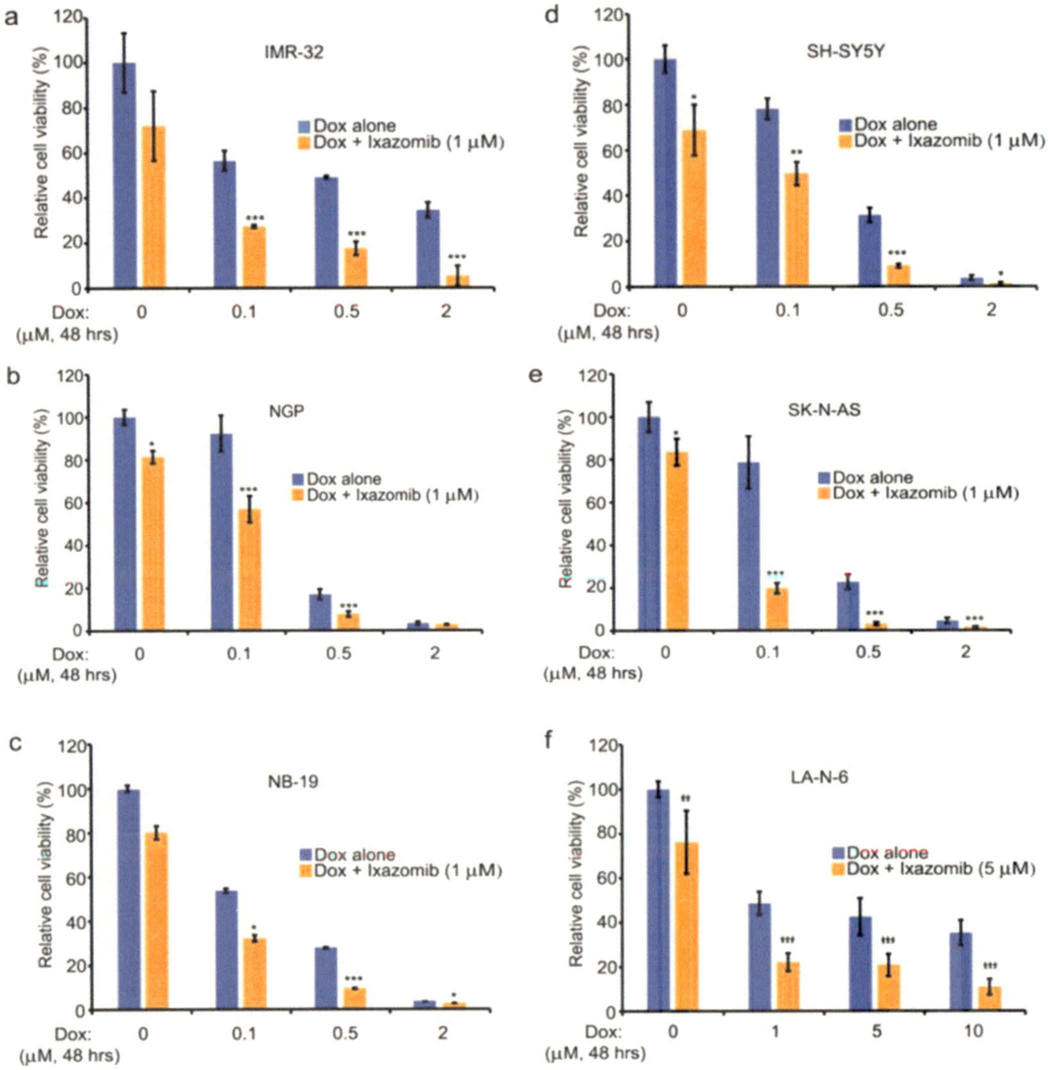

Figure 4. Cell viability results after Dox plus ixazomib (1 or 5 μM) for 48 h; data showed that Ixazomib enhances dox-induced cytotoxicity in different types of Neuroblastoma cell lines. (a–f) IMR-32 (a) NGP (b) NB-19 (c) SH-SY5Y (d) SK-N-AS (e) and LA-N-6 (f) cells were seeded in 96-well plates (Li et al., 2016) [59].

4. Clinical trials for neuroblastoma

Since epigenetic dysregulation is a fundamental process underlying the pathogenesis of pediatric brain tumors, the use of epigenetic modifiers is currently under evaluation in the early phase of clinical trials. Epigenetic modifiers FDA approved mainly comprise two classes of agents: HDACs inhibitors (Vorinostat, Romidepsin, and Valproic Acid) and DNA methylation inhibitors (5-azacytidine and Deoxyazacytidine (Decitabine)).

In November 2015, a phase I trial aiming to test the toxicity of Vorinostat in combination with Isotretinoin and to see how well they work in treating patients with high risk of refractory or recurrent neuroblastoma has been completed. Results showed that Vorinostat may stop the growth of tumor cells by blocking some of the enzymes needed for cell growth; in addition, Isotretinoin may help Vorinostat to work better making tumor cells more sensitive to the drug. The deduction aroused from results has been that Vorinostat together with Isotretinoin may be an effective treatment for neuroblastoma [61]. Simultaneously, another study tested the efficacy of Vorinostat and Iobenguane I 131 (131-I MIBG) to treat patients with resistant or relapsed neuroblastoma. The results demonstrated that the association of Vorinostat together with 131-I MIBG kills more tumor cells, since 131-I MIBG is a radioactive drugs which carry radiation directly to the tumor cells [62, 63].

A phase I study on Decitabine with Doxorubicin in children with neuroblastoma, and other solid tumors, revealed dose-limiting hematologic toxicities which were experienced by children [64]. It is still controversial whether drug toxicity and response rates to HDAC and DNA methylation inhibitors are strictly determined by the somatic tumor genotype or whether heritable germline factors may also contribute to the final outcomes [65]. Thus, it will be crucial to establish the optimal dose and treatment schedule of available drugs, especially considering heavily pretreated patients. To this end, biomarkers of drug efficacy should be used to ascertain whether pharmacological agents, such as epigenetic modifiers, have the predicted biologic effect. Subsequently, tissue availability should be essential for pathologic assessment of the response whenever new epigenetically targeted agents are introduced into the clinical setting.

Currently, a cohort observational study is ongoing and still recruiting participants at the St. Jude Children's Research Hospital of Memphis, Tennessee (US). The aim of the study is to characterize the molecular, cellular, and genetic properties of primary and metastatic neuroblastoma, osteosarcoma, and other solid tumors. The isolated cells will be used for gene expression analysis, genomic analysis by single nucleotide polymorphism (SNP), comparative genomic hybridization, and next-generation sequencing. Epigenetic studies will be also performed investigating at the methylation profile of these cells [66].

At present, there are approximately 500 ongoing clinical trials for neuroblastoma using different therapeutic strategies [67], and only two of these comprise an epigenetic approach [68]. By contrast, as regard the use of proteasome inhibitors there are approximately 80 and 130 ongoing clinical trials, respectively, on Ixazomib and Carfilzomib, to test the side effects and best dose in different cancer conditions [69], but none of these is exclusive for patients affected by neuroblastoma disease [70].

5. Taking advantage of neuroblastoma cells: versatile model for neurobiology studies

The ability to produce *in vitro* cultures of neuronal cells has been crucial for the understanding of central nervous system (CNS) function regulation. The neuronal cell ability to proliferate, as well as to differentiate, makes them an excellent *in vitro* system for several studies. The secondary cell lines derived from neuronal tumors are usually immortalized; they have the advantage to grow easily, to give unlimited proliferation *in vitro*, and to minimize variability between cultures. Cell lines are often induced to display a more neuronal phenotype by manipulations of the culture conditions, for example, through the addition of specific differentiation factors such as retinoic acid.

Neuroblastoma SH-SY5Y cells retain the ability to differentiate into neuronal cell types by all-trans-retinoic acid treatment which causes substantial alterations in the abundance of distinct G protein subunits [71]. In this regard, they have been used to examine the relationships between proliferation, differentiation, and apoptosis and this feature has been useful for the development of therapeutic strategies.

Neuroblastoma cells are extensively used for testing neurotoxicity of putative drugs, and also for understanding neuroplasticity phenomena, such as those evoked by the exposure of drugs of abuse. In particular, studies conducted in human neuroblastoma SH-SY5Y cells demonstrated that ethanol exposure influences epigenetic regulation through histone acetylation, hence regulating DNA transcription at specific portions of the genome [72]. Drugs of abuse have also been associated with proteasome inhibition which seems to be a key player in epigenetic mechanisms underlying the accumulation of oxidatively damaged histones [73]. In this frame, recent finding showed that ethanol exposure reduced intracellular 20S proteasome chymotrypsin-like activity in SH-SY5Y cells [74], in agreement with findings obtained in liver and brain demonstrating that ethanol decreased proteasome activity by interfering with 20S-CP (core particle) and 19S-RP (regulatory particle) assembly [75, 76]. By contrast, cocaine has been reported to exert an opposite effect on the 20S proteasome, since the chymotrypsin-like activity [74] increases.

Although some studies failed to demonstrate the correlation between the increased risk of neuroblastoma in offspring and parental alcohol or tobacco use [77, 78], neuroblastoma cell cultures currently represent a useful tool for the study of neuroplasticity phenomena.

6. Highlights and conclusions

In the last decades, a great variety of novel therapeutic strategies have become available for cancer. These therapies often are very specific and effective only in subsets of cancer patients, thus increasing the needs for the clinician to choose specific therapeutic strategy. This situation exerts a notable impact on the methods in diagnostic tumor pathology, since it requires precise tumor characterization to support the clinical management of the individual case. In this frame, epigenetic changes are important for the initiation and progression of cancers, including neuroblastoma. New insights into tumor biology are driving the development of novel therapeutic approaches which include small-molecule inhibitors as well as epigenetic approaches. The reversible nature of epigenetic modifications, the better knowledge of mechanisms underlying these changes and the consequent alterations of regulatory networks, may provide an interesting opportunity for the development of clinically relevant therapeutics. In particular, histone changes and DNA methylation are fundamental biological processes and they seem to be promising candidates for pharmacological manipulation with encouraging therapeutic advantages.

Acknowledgements

This work was supported by the laboratory of Cellular and Molecular Neuropharmacology from Alma Mater Studiorum, University of Bologna.

Appendices

Histone	H (H1, H2A, H2B, H3, H4)
K	lysine
R	arginine
S	serine
SWI/SNF	switching defective/sucrose non-fermenting
ISWI	imitation-switch
Mi-2/NuRD	Mi-2/nucleosome remodeling and histone deacetylation
INO80	inositol 80
PTMs	posttranslational modifications
HATs	histone acetyl-transferases
HDACs	histone deacetylases
tri-methylation	me3
PRMT1	protein arginine methyltransferases
5mC	5-methylcytosine
DNMTs	DNA methyltransferases (DNMT1, DNMT3A, DNMT3A2, DNMT3B, DNMT3B1, DNMT3B3, DNMT3B7)
NSCs	neural stem cells
ESCs	embryonic stem cells
TSP-1	angiogenesis inhibitor thrombospondin-1
Dox	Doxorubicin
NF-κB	Nuclear factor kappa B transcription factor
IκBα	Nuclear factor kappa B inhibitor, alpha
CP	proteasome core particle
RP	proteasome regulatory particle
PRMT1	protein arginine methyltransferases family 1
CASZ1	zinc-finger transcription factor castor (human castor gene)
SNP	Single nucleotide polymorphism

Author details

Francesca Felicia Caputi*, Sanzio Candeletti and Patrizia Romualdi

*Address all correspondence to: francesca.caputi3@unibo.it

Department of Pharmacy and Biotechnology, Alma Mater Studiorum—University of Bologna, Bologna, Italy

References

[1] Berger SL. The complex language of chromatin regulation during transcription. Nature. 2007;**447**:407-412

[2] Memorial University, Faculty of Science - Biology [internet]. Available from: http://www.mun.ca/biology/desmid/brian/BIOL2060/BIOL2060-18/18_21.jpg [Accessed: April 14, 2017]

[3] Kasten MM, Clapier CR, Cairns BR. SnapShot: Chromatin remodeling: SWI/SNF. Cell. 2011;**144:**e311

[4] Yadon AN, Tsukiyama T. SnapShot: Chromatin remodeling: ISWI. Cell. 2011;**144**:453-453.e1

[5] Lai AY, Wade PA. Cancer biology and NuRD: A multifaceted chromatin remodelling complex. Nature Review Cancer. 2011;**11**:588-596

[6] Bao Y, Shen X. SnapShot: Chromatin remodeling: INO80 and SWR1. Cell. 2011;**144**: 158-158e2

[7] Helming KC, Wang X, Roberts CW. Vulnerabilities of mutant SWI/SNF complexes in cancer. Cancer Cell. 2014;**26**:309-317

[8] Kahali B, Yu J, Marquez SB, Thompson KW, Liang SY, Lu L, Reisman D. The silencing of the SWI/SNF subunit and anticancer gene BRM in Rhabdoid tumors. Oncotarget. 2014;**5**:3316-3332

[9] Xie C, Fu L, Xie L, Liu N, Li Q. Rsf-1 overexpression serves as a prognostic marker in human hepatocellular carcinoma. Tumour Biology. 2014;**35**:7595-7601

[10] Liu S, Dong Q, Wang E. Rsf-1 overexpression correlates with poor prognosis and cell proliferation in colon cancer. Tumour Biology. 2012;**33**:1485-1491

[11] Legube G, Trouche D. Regulating histone acetyltransferases and deacetylases. EMBO Reproduction. 2003;**4**:944-947

[12] Seto E, Yoshida M. Erasers of histone acetylation: The histone deacetylase enzymes. Cold Spring Harbour Perspectives in Biology. 2014;**6**:a018713

[13] Seidel C, Schnekenburger M, Dicato M, Diederich M. Histone deacetylase modulators provided by mother nature. Genes & Nutrition. 2012;**7**:357-367

[14] Bedford MT, Clarke SG. Protein arginine methylation in mammals: Who, what, and why. Molecular Cell. 2009;**33**:1-13

[15] Kouzarides, T. Chromatin modifications and their function. Cell. 2007;**128**:693-705

[16] Zhang Y, Reinberg D. Transcription regulation by histone methylation: Interplay between different covalent modifications of the core histone tails. Genes & Development. 2001;**15**: 2343-2360

[17] Rice JC, Briggs SD, Ueberheide B, Barber CM, Shabanowitz J, Hunt DF, Shinkai Y, Allis CD. Histone methyltransferases direct different degrees of methylation to define distinct chromatin domains. Molecular Cell. 2003;**12**:1591-1598

[18] Ehrlich M, Lacey M. DNA hypomethylation and hemimethylation in cancer. Advances in Experimental Medicine and Biology. 2013;**754**:31-56

[19] Kinney SR, Pradhan S. Regulation of expression and activity of DNA (cytosine-5) methyltransferases in mammalian cells. Progress in Molecular Biology and Translational Science. 2011;**101**:311-333

[20] Song J, Teplova M, Ishibe-Murakami S, Patel DJ. Structure-based mechanistic insights into DNMT1- mediated maintenance DNA methylation. Science. 2011;**335**:709-712

[21] Sharma S, Kelly TK, Jones PA. Epigenetics in cancer. Carcinogenesis. 2010;**31**:27-36

[22] Wu Y, Strawn E, Basir Z, Halverson G, Guo SW. Aberrant expression of deoxyribonucleic acid methyltransferases DNMT1, DNMT3A, and DNMT3B in women with endometriosis. Fertility and Sterility. 2007;**87**:24-32

[23] Berman BP, Weisenberger DJ, Aman JF, Hinoue T, Ramjan Z, Liu Y, Noushmehr H, Lange CP, van Dijk CM, Tollenaar RA, Den Berg DV, Laird PW. Regions of focal DNA hypermethylation and long-range hypomethylation in colorectal cancer coincide with nuclear lamina-associated domains. Nature Genetics. 2012;**44**:40-46

[24] Hur K, Cejas P, Feliu J, Moreno-Rubio J, Burgos E, Boland CR, Goel A. Hypomethylation of long interspersed nuclear element-1 (LINE-1) leads to activation of proto-oncogenes in human colorectal cancer metastasis. Gut. 2014;**63**:635-646

[25] Figueroa ME, Abdel-Wahab O, Lu C, Ward PS, Patel J, Shih A, Li Y, Bhagwat N, Vasanthakumar A, Fernandez HF, Tallman MS, Sun Z, Wolniak K, Peeters JK, Liu W, Choe SE, Fantin VR, Paietta E, Löwenberg B, Licht JD, Godley LA, Delwel R, Valk PJM, Thompson CB, Levine RL, Melnick A. Leukemic IDH1 and IDH2 mutations result in a hypermethylation phenotype, disrupt TET2 function, and impair hematopoietic differentiation. Cancer Cell. 2010;**18**:553-567

[26] Rideout WM, 3rd, Coetzee GA, Olumi AF, Jones PA. 5-Methylcytosine as an endogenous mutagen in the human LDL receptor and p53 genes. Science 1990;**249**:1288-1290

[27] Pfeifer GP, Tang M, Denissenko MF. Mutation hotspots and DNA methylation. Current Topics in Microbiology and Immunology. 2000;**249**:1-19

[28] Pugh TJ, Morozova O, Attiyeh EF, Asgharzadeh S, Wei JS, Auclair D, Carter SL, Cibulskis K, Hanna M, Kiezun A, et al. The genetic landscape of high-risk neuroblastoma. Nature Genetics. 2013;**45**:279-284

[29] Burney MJ, Johnston C, Wong KY, et al. An epigenetic signature of developmental potential in neural stem cells and early neurons. Stem Cells. 2013;**31**:1868-1880

[30] Delaval K, Feil R. Epigenetic regulation of mammalian genomic imprinting. Current Opinion in Genetics Development. 2004;**14**:188-195

[31] Margueron R, Trojer P, Reinberg D. The key to development: interpreting the histone code? Current Opinion in Genetics Development. 2005;**15**:163-176

[32] Bernstein BE, Mikkelsen TS, Xie X. et al. A bivalent chromatin structure marks key developmental genes in embryonic stem cells. Cell. 2006;**125**:315-326

[33] Okano H, Temple S. Cell types to order: Temporal specification of CNS stem cells. Current Opinion in Neurobiology. 2009;**19**:112-119

[34] Sharma SV, Lee DY, Li B, Quinlan MP, Takahashi F, Maheswaran S, McDermott U, Azizian N, Zou L, Fischbach MA, et al. A chromatin-mediated reversible drug-tolerant state in cancer cell subpopulations. Cell. 2010;**141**:69-80

[35] Baylin SB, Jones PA. Epigenetic determinants of cancer. Cold Spring Harbour in Perspective Biology. 2016;**8**pii:a019505

[36] Okano M, Bell DW, Haber DA, Li E. DNA methyltransferases Dnmt3a and Dnmt3b are essential for de novo methylation and mammalian development. Cell. 1999;**99**:247-257

[37] Goll MG, Bestor TH. Eukaryotic cytosine methyltransferases. Annual Review in Biochemistry. 2005;**74**:481-514

[38] Bestor T, Laudano A, Mattaliano R, Ingram V. Cloning and sequencing of a cDNA encoding DNA methyltransferase of mouse cells. The carboxyl-terminal domain of the mammalian enzymes is related to bacterial restriction methyltransferases. Journal of Molecular Biology. 1988;**203**:971-983

[39] Okano M, Xie S, Li E. Cloning and characterization of a family of novel mammalian DNA (cytosine-5) methyltransferases. Nature Genetics. 1998;**19**:219-220

[40] Lei H, Oh SP, Okano M, Jüttermann R, Goss KA, Jaenisch R, Li E. De novo DNA cytosine methyltransferase activities in mouse embryonic stem cells. Development. 1996;**122**: 3195-3205

[41] Chen T, Ueda Y, Dodge JE, Wang Z, Li E. Establishment and maintenance of genomic methylation patterns in mouse embryonic stem cells by Dnmt3a and Dnmt3b. Molecule & Cell Biology. 2003;**23**:5594-5605

[42] Hatziapostolou M, Iliopoulos D. Epigenetic aberrations during oncogenesis. Cellular and Molecular Life Sciences. 2011;**68**:1681-1702

[43] Esteller M. Cancer epigenomics: DNA methylomes and histone-modification maps. Nature Review Genetics. 2007;**8**:286-298

[44] Liu Z, Yang X, Li Z, McMahon C, Sizer C, Barenboim-Stapleton L, Bliskovsky V, Mock B, Ried T, London WB, Maris J, Khan J, Thiele CJ. CASZ1, a candidate tumor-suppressor gene, suppresses neuroblastoma tumor growth through reprogramming gene expression. Cell Death Differentiation. 2011;**18**:1174-1183

[45] Fransson S, Martinsson T, Ejeskär K. Neuroblastoma tumors with favorable and unfavorable outcomes: Significant differences in mRNA expression of genes mapped at 1p36.2. Genes, Chromosomes and Cancer. 2007;**46**:45-52

[46] Carén H, Ejeskär K, Fransson S, Hesson L, Latif F, Sjöberg RM, Krona C, Martinsson T. A cluster of genes located in 1p36 are down-regulated in neuroblastomas with poor prognosis, but not due to CpG island methylation. Molecular Cancer. 2005;**4**:10

[47] Lee ER, Murdoch FE, Fritsch MK. High histone acetylation and decreased polycomb repressive complex 2 member levels regulate gene specific transcriptional changes during early embryonic stem cell differentiation induced by retinoic acid. Stem Cells. 2007;**25**:2191-2199

[48] Yang QW, Liu S, Tian, Y, et al. Methylation-associated silencing of the thrombospondin-1 gene in human neuroblastoma. Cancer Research. 2003;**63**:6299-6310

[49] Breit S, Ashman K, Wilting J, Rossler J, Hatzi E, Fotsis T, Schweigerer L. The N-*myc* oncogene in human neuroblastoma cells: Down-regulation of an angiogenesis inhibitor identified as Activin A. Cancer Research. 2000;**60**:4596-4601

[50] Davidoff AM, Leary MA, Ng CY, Vanin EF. Gene therapy-mediated expression by tumor cells of the angiogenesis inhibitor flk-1 results in inhibition of neuroblastoma growth *in vivo*. Journal of Pediatric Surgery. 2001;**36**:30-36

[51] Saito Y, Kanai Y, Sakamoto M, Saito H, Ishii H, Hirohashi S. Overexpression of a splice variant of DNA methyltransferase 3b, DNMT3b4, associated with DNA hypomethylation on pericentromeric satellite regions during human hepatocarcinogenesis. Proceedings of the National Academy of Sciences United States of America. 2002;**99**:10060-10065

[52] Ostler KR, Yang Q, Looney TJ, Zhang L, Vasanthakumar A, Tian Y, Kocherginsky M, Raimondi SL, DeMaio JG, Salwen HR, Gu S, Chlenski A, Naranjo A, Gill A, Peddinti R, Lahn BT, Cohn SL, Godley LA. Truncated DNMT3B isoform DNMT3B7 suppresses growth, induces differentiation, and alters DNA methylation in human neuroblastoma. Cancer Research. 2012;**72**:4714-4723

[53] Jordan CT, Guzman ML, Noble M. Cancer stem cells. New England Journal of Medicine. 2006;**355**:1253-1261

[54] Eyler CE, Rich JN. Survival of the fittest: Cancer stem cells in therapeutic resistance and angiogenesis. Journal of Clinical Oncology. 2008;**26**:2839-2845

[55] Rivankar S. An overview of doxorubicin formulations in cancer therapy. Journal of Cancer Research Therapy. 2014;**10**:853-858

[56] Ku JM, Kim SR, Hong SH, Choi HS, Seo HS, Shin YC, Ko SG. Cucurbitacin D induces cell cycle arrest and apoptosis by inhibiting STAT3 and NF-κB signaling in doxorubicin-resistant human breast carcinoma (MCF7/ADR) cells. Molecular and Cell Biochemistry. 2015;**409**:33-43

[57] Rajkumar SV, Richardson PG, Hideshima T, Anderson KC. Proteasome inhibition as a novel therapeutic target in human cancer. Journal of Clinical Oncology. 2005;**23**:630-639

[58] Palombella VJ, Rando OJ, Goldberg AL, Maniatis T. The ubiquitin-proteasome pathway is required for processing the NF-kappa B1 precursor protein and the activation of NF-kappa B. Cell. 1994;**78**:773-785

[59] Li H, Chen Z, Hu T, Wang L, Yu Y., Zhao, Y, Sun W, Guan S, Pang JC, Woodfield SE, Liu Q, Yang J. Novel proteasome inhibitor ixazomib sensitizes neuroblastoma cells to doxorubicin treatment. Scientific Report. 2016;**30**:6:34397

[60] Guan S, Zhao Y, Lu J, Yu Y, Sun W, Mao X, Chen Z, Xu X, Pan J, Sun S, Yang J. Second-generation proteasome inhibitor carfilzomib sensitizes neuroblastoma cells to doxorubicin-induced apoptosis. Oncotarget. 2016;**7**:75914-75925

[61] National Cancer Institute (NIH) [Internet]. Available from: www.cancer.gov/clinicaltrials; NCT01208454. [Accessed: 14-April-2017]

[62] National Cancer Institute (NIH) [Internet]. Available from: www.cancer.gov/clinicaltrials;NCT01019850. [Accessed: 14-April-2017]

[63] Matthay KK, George RE, Yu AL. Promising therapeutic targets in neuroblastoma. Clinical Cancer Research. 2012;**18**:2740-2753

[64] George RE, Lahti JM, Adamson PC, Zhu K, Finkelstein D, Ingle AM, et al. Phase I study of decitabine with doxorubicin and cyclophosphamide in children with neuroblastoma and other solid tumors: A Children's Oncology Group study. Pediatric Blood & Cancer. 2010;**55**:629-638

[65] Pinto N, Cohn SL, Dolan ME. Using germline genomics to individualize pediatric cancer treatments. Clinical Cancer Research. 2012;**18**:2791-2800

[66] National Cancer Institute (NIH) [Internet]. Available from:www.cancer.gov/clinicaltrials; NCT01050296. [Accessed: 14-April-2017]

[67] National Cancer Institute (NIH) [Internet]. Available from: https://clinicaltrials.gov/ct2/results?term=neuroblastoma+&Search=Search [Accessed: 14-April-2017]

[68] National Cancer Institute (NIH) [Internet]. Available from: https://clinicaltrials.gov/ct2/results?term=neuroblastoma+and+epigenetic+&Search=Search. [Accessed: 14-April-2017]

[69] National Cancer Institute (NIH) [Internet]. Available from: https://clinicaltrials.gov/ct2/results?term=ixazomib&Search=Search. [Accessed: 14-April-2017]

[70] National Cancer Institute (NIH) [Internet]. Available from: https://clinicaltrials.gov/ct2/results?term=ixazomib+AND+neuroblastoma&Search=Search. [Accessed: 14-April-2017]

[71] Ammer H, Schulz R. Retinoic acid-induced differentiation of human neuroblastoma SH-SY5Y cells is associated with changes in the abundance of G proteins. Journal of Neurochemistry. 1994;**62**:1310-1318

[72] D'Addario C, Johansson S, Candeletti S, Romualdi P, Ögren SO, Terenius L, Ekström TJ. Ethanol and acetaldehyde exposure induces specific epigenetic modifications in the prodynorphin gene promoter in a human neuroblastoma cell line. FASEB Journal. 2011;**25**:1069-1075

[73] Bardag-Gorce F. Nuclear effects of ethanol-induced proteasome inhibition in liver cells. World Journal of Gastroenterology. 2009;**15**:1163-1167

[74] Caputi FF, Carboni L, Mazza D, Candeletti S, Romualdi P. Cocaine and ethanol target 26S proteasome activity and gene expression in neuroblastoma cells. Drug and Alcohol Dependence. 2016;**161**:265-275

[75] Donohue Jr TM, Thomes PG. Ethanol-induced oxidant stress modulates hepatic autophagy and proteasome activity. Redox Biology. 2014;**3**:29-39

[76] Erdozain AM, Morentin B, Bedford L, King E, Tooth D, Brewer C, Wayne D, Johnson L, Gerdes HK, Wigmore P, Callado LF, Carter WG. Alcohol-related brain damage in humans. PLoS One. 2014;**9**:e93586

[77] Yang Q, Olshan AF, Bondy ML, Shah NR, Pollock BH, Seeger RC, Look AT, Cohn SL. Parental smoking and alcohol consumption and risk of neuroblastoma. Cancer Epidemiology, Biomarkers & Prevention. 2000;**9**:967-972

[78] Norman MA, Holly EA, Ahn DK, Preston-Martin S, Mueller BA, Bracci PM. Prenatal exposure to tobacco smoke and childhood brain tumors: Results from the United States West Coast childhood brain tumor study. Cancer Epidemiology, Biomarkers & Prevention.1996;**5**:127-133

Considerations for the Development of Innovative Therapies Against Aggressive Neuroblastoma: Immunotherapy and Twist1 Targeting

Tala Shekarian and Sandrine Valsesia-Wittmann

Additional information is available at the end of the chapter

http://dx.doi.org/10.5772/intechopen.70000

Abstract

Neuroblastoma (NB) is one of the major challenges of pediatric oncology with a 5-year survival rate of less than 40% despite intense therapy. The aggressiveness of the disease has been recently correlated to the degree of myeloid cells infiltrating the tumor. Together with the tumor cells and immunosuppressive cytokines (e.g., IL-10 and TGF-β), these cells hamper the generation of an efficient antitumor immune response and, therefore, favor tumor growth and metastasis. Novel therapeutic approaches are designed to target immune cells instead of cancer cells. To improve their efficacy, recent cancer immunotherapy strategies have focused on the depletion, blockade, or reprogramming of these tolerogenic immune effectors. Therefore, the principal clinical challenge is currently to identify therapeutic strategies which could overcome the primary and secondary resistances to these cancer immunotherapies. In this review, we discuss the dialogue of immune microenvironment of neuroblastoma and the immunotherapeutic strategies to cure neuroblastoma.

Keywords: immunotherapy, immune checkpoint modulators, microenvironment, inflammation, *TWIST1*

1. Introduction

Our immune system is continuously monitoring our tissues and recognizes the abnormal cancer cells to kill them. The immune cells originate from hematopoietic stem cells inside the bone marrow that give birth to two different lineages: the myeloid and lymphoid progenitor cells. The different populations derived from myeloid progenitor cells are monocytes, macrophages, neutrophils, basophils, eosinophils, erythrocytes, dendritic cells (DC), and megakaryocytes

INTECH
open science | open minds

© 2017 The Author(s). Licensee InTech. This chapter is distributed under the terms of the Creative Commons Attribution License (http://creativecommons.org/licenses/by/3.0), which permits unrestricted use, distribution, and reproduction in any medium, provided the original work is properly cited. (cc) BY (or platelets). The population driven from lymphoid progenitor cells is T and B lymphocytes, natural killer (NK) cells, and other innate lymphoid cells. These different populations are the principal actors of innate and adaptive immune system. The innate immunity populations include the natural killer cells, granulocytic cells, such as neutrophil, and antigen presenting cells (APC), such as DC and macrophages. These cells provide the first line of self-defense against foreign pathogens as well as cellular damages and cancers. The innate immune response is very rapid but has no antigen specificity and immunological memory. In contrast to the innate immune response, adaptive immune responses are highly specific to the particular antigen and provide a long-lasting protection through induction of memory. The two populations of adaptive immunity are T lymphocyte populations (T helper and cytotoxic T cells) and B lymphocytes (plasma cells which are capable to secrete the antibodies).

The fact that tumors arise from self-tissues expressing antigens which induced immune tolerance implies the lack of immunogenicity and lack of immune control of the tumor. Latter based on different studies, the concept of immune editing emerged [1]. This process contains three phases: elimination, equilibrium, and escape. Elimination is the classical concept of immune surveillance, whereas the Darwinian natural selection of tumor variant developing the mutations which make them resistant to immune attacks occurs in the equilibrium phase. This process can lead to immune escape of immune resistant tumor variants and the formation of clinically apparent tumors [2]. It is now accepted that the immune system has a primary role in the prevention of tumors.

In high-risk neuroblastoma (HRNB), amplification of MYCN oncogene leads to an important oncogenic stress that normally drives to the induction of a program allowing the elimination of proliferating cells by cell death, apoptosis, or replicative senescence.

Usually, apoptotic or necrotic bodies are uptaken by antigen presenting cells (APC) allowing their elimination by the immune system leading to an adaptive immune response. Therefore, immune editing is a crucial step in tumor development. However, neuroblastoma (NB) is a pediatric tumor and from an immunological point of view, children age clearly determines the status and capacities of an adaptive immune response. Children less than 1 year of age with immature immune system, with innate cells preferentially, have better prognosis than children more than 1 year of age with a more mature immune system. These paradoxical observations reflect the functional duality of immune system harboring both the antitumoral and protumoral abilities.

Interestingly, metastatic tumors diagnosed in children at age ≥18 months had higher expression of inflammation-related genes than those in patients diagnosed at age <18 months. These data suggest that these inflammatory cells in the tumor microenvironment may contribute to the clinical metastatic neuroblastoma phenotype and reveal a novel rational for immunotherapy of neuroblastoma (NB) [3].

2. Immunotherapy of neuroblastoma

Checkpoint inhibitors, such as ipilimumab (anti-CTLA4) or pembrolizumab (anti-PD1), demonstrated spectacular benefit in some adult cancers, but lack of activity in pediatric cancers, likely due to the rarity of neoantigens [4]. Neoantigens are uniquely present on the tumor and not expressed by normal tissue, in contrast to different molecules overexpressed on tumors that are also present on normal prenatal or postnatal tissues, which induce immune tolerance. In fact, many adult tumors arise in response to environmentally mediated genotoxic damage and bear large numbers of mutations. In contrast, pediatric tumors typically display few mutations but mostly translocations or gene amplifications. In NB, MYCN amplification, activating mutations, or rearrangements of *ALK* (observed in 8–10% of sporadic tumors) preexist in prenatal tissues and might be responsible for immune tolerance [5]. Therefore, NB (and others pediatric cancers) can be compared with resistant to immune checkpoint inhibitors in adult cancers and need to be treated as such. First, while pediatric tumors demonstrate low mutation burdens at diagnosis, increases in mutation frequency can be enhanced after exposure to chemotherapy or radiotherapy [6, 7]. In addition to increase neoantigens, radiation may increase immune response to checkpoint blockade as localized radiation along with checkpoint blockade resulted in an abscopal effect with regression of metastatic lesions outside of the radiation field [8]. Using agents that induce tumor cell death or tissue differentiation might lead to release or expression of new tumor-associated antigens (TAA) or differentiation antigens. Therefore, combining checkpoint inhibitors with agents that augment innate and/or adaptive immunity could provide effective antitumor responses in children despite low inherent immunogenicity [9].

Synthetic immunotherapies, such as monoclonal antibodies (Mabs) and chimeric antigen receptor (CAR) T cells, harbor such characteristics. This is probably one reason of their impressive effects against childhood cancers in general. The only clinically available mAbs in neuroblastoma cells is dinutuximab, a chimeric, human-murine, anti-disialoganglioside GD2 overexpressed on NB tumors. Dinutuximab was approved in combination with granulocyte/monocyte-colony stimulating factor (GM-CSF), aldesleukin (interleukin-2 [IL-2]), and isotretinoin (13-cis-retinoic acid [RA]) for maintenance treatment of patients with high-risk neuroblastoma who respond at least to first-line multimodality therapy [10]. In phase III trials, dinutuximab increased 2-year event-free survival (EFS) and overall survival (OS) compared to standard treatment. It was shown that major mechanism of action of dinutuximab passes though the induction of antibody-dependent cell-mediated cytotoxicity (ADCC) and complement-dependent cytotoxicity (CDC) leading to tumor cells lysis and TAA release [11]. Therefore, combination of dinutuximab with immune checkpoint inhibitors, such as anti-PD1/PDL1 Mabs, might increase effective adaptive antitumor immune response leading to better survival. Since serious adverse reactions have been reported with the dinutuximab-containing regimen, with infusion reactions and neuropathy prompting the Food and Drug Agency (FDA) to issue boxed warnings, this combination could be a very promising issue.

Another promising way to stimulate immune system consists in the development of bispecific antibody targeting GD2 and CD3 expressed on T cells. The idea to bridge activated T cells (ATC) to GD2-positive neuroblastomas provides preclinical rationale for immunotherapy using this bispecific antibody in children with neuroblastoma [12].

Another novel approach recently developed to improve the current anti-GD2 immunotherapy is based on NK cell stimulation using Toll-like receptor (TLR) activated plasmacytoid dendritic cells (pDCs). NK activation by pDCs led to a NK-cell phenotype characterized by increased surface expression of tumor necrosis factor-related apoptosis-inducing ligand

(TRAIL), CD69 on CD56dim cytotoxic cells, and strong interferon-γ production. These data suggest that children with HRNB may benefit from NK-cell stimulation by activated pDCs to increase NK-cell lytic functions against NB cells [13].

In fact, NK cells impact on the normal immune surveillance of HRNB. Quantification of serum concentration of soluble B7-H6, ligand of NKp30 activation molecule, correlated with the downregulation of NKp30, bone marrow metastasis, and chemoresistance [14]. Thus, interaction between NKp30 and B7-H6 may contribute to neuroblastoma immunosurveillance and both NKp30 expression on circulating NK cells and the serum concentration of soluble B7-H6 may represent biomarkers for risk stratification [14].

Although adoptive transfer of T cells expressing chimeric antigen receptors (CARs) targeting hematopoietic lineage demonstrated impressive response in chemorefractory pediatric patients, in solid tumors, lack of efficacy seems multifactorial and includes the suppressive tumor microenvironment [15, 16].

Pule et al. reported partial response in patients with refractory neuroblastoma using first-generation GD2-CAR (e.g., TCR zeta signaling endodomains without additional costimulation) incorporating the scFv shared with dinutuximab [17]. Efforts to add both CD28 and OX40 as costimulatory domains were disappointing with no improved objective response [18].

CD171 (L1-CAM) is another abundant cell surface molecule expressed on neuroblastomas, which is detectable at the diagnosis and relapse time independently on patient clinical risk. The CE7R CAR targeting CD171 demonstrated activation of tumor cell lysis and Th1 cytokine production [19, 20]. Infusion of autologous CD8(+) cytolytic T lymphocyte clones coexpressing CE7R and the selection suicide expression enzyme HyTK in children with recurrent/refractory neuroblastoma was the first-in-humans pilot study that set the stage for clinical trials employing adoptive transfer in the context of minimal residual disease. No overt toxicities to tissues known to express L1-cell adhesion molecule (e.g., central nervous system, adrenal medulla, and sympathetic ganglia) were observed.

Finally, a large panel of primarily resected neuroblastoma samples demonstrated expression of the cancer-testis antigen (NY-ESO-1) in 23% of the samples. NY-ESO-1 is expressed by many solid tumors and has limited expression by mature somatic tissues, making it a highly attractive target for tumor immunotherapy. Transgenic TCR (tTCRs combined with HLA-A2+ neuroblastoma cell lines) targeting NY-ESO-1 has been shown to slow the progression of both local and disseminated disease, and significantly enhanced animal survival providing rational for therapeutic option for patients with neuroblastoma [21].

Again, as proposed for therapeutic Mabs, the combination of CAR T cells with immune checkpoint modulators could bring a profit in terms of antitumoral response and remain to be evaluated.

Recent studies have shown that MYCN nonamplified metastatic neuroblastomas have higher infiltration of Tumor Asociated Macrophages (TAM) myeloid CD163+ cells than locoregional tumors. Macrophage-colony stimulating factor (M-CSF) or colony stimulating factor (CSF-1) is known to be essential for the differentiation and survival of these myeloid cells [22]. It is associated with poor survival in various human cancer and CSF-1R (CSF-1 receptor) targeting strategies have been explored [23]. In NB, it has been shown that CSF-1R+ myeloid cells predict poor survival in patients and, as a consequence, combining CSF-1R inhibitor (BLZ945) with PD-1/PD-L1 blocking agents induce robust antitumor effects against established aggressive tumors in the TH-*MYCN* murine neuroblastoma model [24].

Cytokine-induced killer (CIK) cells, immune effector cells that have the properties of T lymphocyte and NK cells, capable to recognize malignant cells in the absence of Major Histocompatibility Complex (MHC), also have provided encouraging results in clinical studies. IL-15-activated CIK cells have revealed synergistic antitumor effects in combination with standard therapy and higher toxicity in comparison with IL-2-stimulated NK cells [25].

3. New prospects in immunotherapy

A very promising therapy currently in development in adult cancer consists in the combination of oncolytic viruses (OVs) with immune checkpoint inhibitors. Oncolytic viruses can infect cancer cells and induce cell death to produce the new viruses. Some oncolytic viruses, such as parvovirus, reovirus, Newcastle disease virus (NDV), mumps virus, or Moloney leukemia virus, have natural preference to replicate into cancer cells leading to the destruction of the cells [26]. Viruses such as measles virus, adenovirus, vesicular stomatitis virus (VSV), vaccinia virus (VV), and herpes simplex virus (HSV) can be engineered to confer them cancer specificity [26]. Some were engineered to directly target unique cell surface receptors expressed by cancer cells such as adenovirus to target CAR [27] and measles virus to express a single-chain antibody that recognizes carcinoembryonic antigen (CEA) [28]. Others are deficient viruses like E1B mutant adenovirus which preferentially replicate in p53 inactivated cells [29].

There are already two engineered OVs approved in clinic in adults: E1B-deleted adenovirus and talimogene laherparepvec virus (T-VEC). T-VEC is based on herpes simplex virus type 1 deleted for ICP 34.5 gene (neurovirulence factor), ICP47 (block antigen presentation in HSV infected cell), overexpressed US11 (viral RNA binding proteins), and inserted for GM-SCF [30]. T-VEC is approved by the FDA for the treatment of melanoma [31]. Others are under active development.

Most oncolytic viruses can induce cancer cell death and directly eliminate tumor cells but they also initiate systemic immune responses through different mechanisms such as inducing an immunogenic cell death, releasing danger-associated molecular patterns (DAMPs) and tumor-associated antigens (TAA) from virus-infected cells. They also release viral pathogen-associated molecular patterns (PAMPs) contributing APCs maturation that conduct the activation of antigen-specific CD4+ and CD8+ T cell responses. Once activated, CD8+ T cells become cytotoxic effector cells that traffic to tumor sites, where they mediate antitumor immunity upon antigen recognition [32]. Combining checkpoint inhibitors to virotherapies might ultimately prove beneficial for neuroblastoma resistance to immune checkpoint blockade antibody therapy.

4. Twist1 targeted therapy

In correlation with MYCN amplification (NMA), we previously reported that *TWIST1* was constantly overexpressed in neuroblastoma with NMA and highlighted *in vivo* cooperation between *TWIST1* and *MYCN* for primary cells transformation through inhibition of apoptosis and differentiation [33]. Based on different clinical data tumor sets, we demonstrated that *TWIST1* overexpression was associated not only with NMA but also with *MYCN* or *MYC* overexpression and highlighted *TWIST1* as a direct *MYC* transcriptional target [34].

We previously showed that inhibition of *TWIST1* expression restores the apoptotic properties of NB cells overexpressing *MYCN* [33]. Based on the observation that stage 4S NB with higher levels of N-Myc proteins are more prone to spontaneous regression by apoptosis [35] or neuronal differentiation [36], it has been speculated that *MYCN* not only mediates malignant progression, but is also involved in spontaneous regression in favorable NB [37]. We, and others, have demonstrated that inhibition of *MYCN* leads to *MYC* upregulation [38]. For all these reasons, both *MYC* family members have to be simultaneously targeted. Restoration of *MYCN* or *MYC* proapoptotic properties though *TWIST1* inhibition is, therefore, a promising concept.

In many other tumor types, Twist1 has been associated to Epithelial–Mesenchymal Transition (EMT) and cancer stem cell phenotype (CSC) [39]. There are different drugs currently in development targeting the cancer stem cells associated with Twist1 deregulation. Some show promising results from preclinical trials like Salinomycin able to effectively eliminate CSCs and to induce partial clinical regression of heavily pretreated and therapy-resistant cancers [40, 41].

5. TWIST1, MYC, and immune system

Recent papers suggest that oncogenes playing key role in transformation might also play a role in protumoral microenvironment properties [42]. This is true for *TWIST1* since its overexpression was reported correlated with increased vascularization in breast carcinoma [43]. In fact, Twist1 does not directly induce vEGF production by tumor cells but rather chemokines like CCL2 that are attractive for vEGF-producer macrophages. Their homing in tumor microenvironment site and production of vEGF contribute to metastasis [42]. In aggressive NMA neuroblastoma, it was shown that TAMs are correlated to bad prognosis [10]. Macrophages are key players in maintaining the tissue homeostasis, shaping adaptive immune response, inflammation, and tissue repair [44]. In response to signals from the microenvironment, macrophages are polarized into distinct phenotypic subtypes, referred as proinflammatory macrophages M1 and anti-inflammatory M2 subtype [45]. Macrophages that reside within a tumor, often referred as TAMs, display M2-like phenotypes with immunosuppression regulatory functions to support tumor development [46]. Interestingly, it was shown that Twist1 inhibition in tumor cells lead to TAM decrease and vascularization regression. Once more, Twist1 was shown to directly produce immunosuppressive cytokines attracting immunosuppressive Gr1+CD11b+ myeloid-derived suppressive cells (MDSC) in tumor microenvironment that can be reversible after Twist1 inhibition [47]. Therefore, the role of inflammatory cells in tumor microenvironment may contribute to the clinical metastatic neuroblastoma phenotype, improve prognostication, and reveal novel ratio for immunotherapy of neuroblastoma. Interestingly, MYCN has also been recently revealed as the most highly upregulated gene in macrophages upon the treatment of immune suppressive soluble factors that are released from apoptotic cells [48]. Once more, it was shown that inhibition of MYC in macrophages attenuates the protumor function of TAM and suppresses tumor growth [49].

These studies implicate MYC and MYCN as a key player in regulating macrophage functions and suggest that MYC inactivation may suppress tumor growth in a cancer cell-extrinsic manner. Therefore, MYC and MYCN may not only regulate proliferation but also exert immune modulatory functions in macrophages, therefore, on immunosuppressive microenvironment.

Therefore, strategies aiming to inactivate Twist1 and/or Myc proteins might be of interest both on tumor cells survival capacities but mostly in reprogramming the tolerogenic immune effectors within the microenvironment.

For example, Twist1 inhibition might lead from one hand, by inducing tumor cell death or tissue differentiation, to release of tumor-associated antigens or differentiation antigens, and on the other hand, to reprogrammation of inflammatory myeloid cells within tumoral microenvironment. Combination of both events might contribute to efficient destruction of tumors by reactivation of immune system leading to an efficient antitumoral adaptive immune response. Combination with immune checkpoint inhibitors needs to be further analyzed.

6. Conclusion

Despite recent advancement in the understanding of molecular pathways that drive the development of neuroblastoma, insights have not fundamentally changed the therapeutic approach, which still consist in nonspecific, cytotoxic chemotherapy. Chemoresistant and relapse make that neuroblastoma always represents 15% of all pediatric cancer deaths. Innovative treatment approaches are, therefore, needed. Intense efforts are underway to enhance the effectiveness of immunotherapies through combination with agents designed to selectively attack the tumor cells and amplify immune responses.

Based upon the results with dinutuximab, immunotherapy has already demonstrated impressive benefit to children with neuroblastoma. Checkpoint inhibitors administered alone or in combination have not yet been studied in childhood cancer, although they will not be sufficient as single agents. CAR T cells have shown unprecedented results in pediatric hematological cancer but showed limited efficacy in solid tumors to date.

The ultimate goal would rather be to deliver a specific innovative tumor destruction system permitting the release of TAA, and local induction of inflammation, in order to provide immune priming and amplification of the immune response after combination with immune checkpoint modulators. Therefore, strategies that target both tumor cells and microenvironment are focusing interest.

In the race of improving immunotherapy for pediatric cancer, oncolytic viruses might find a very important issue. OVs have many features that make them advantageous for cancer immunotherapy: (1) there is a very low probability for the generation of resistance to virus (not seen so far), because OVs often target multiple oncogenic pathways and induce cytotoxicity in different ways, (2) they are nonpathogenic, replicate, and destroy cancer cells, (3) virus dose in the tumor increases with time due to *in situ* virus amplification, which is opposite to classical drug pharmacokinetics that decreases with time, and (4) OVs can be manipulated to include safety features such as drug and immune sensitivity allowing to control them [50]. Intratumoral delivery of the OVs can be a good strategy to minimize the sequestration of the virus in the spleen and liver as well as antiviral response [26].

Targeting oncogenes that control both tumor cells survival and proliferation and immunosuppressive microenvironment might also bring new hope in the treatment of HNRB. Twist1 and MYC might be suitable for that purpose. Since Twist1 expression is restricted to tumor cells, it represents a very interesting target. Efforts to develop specific drugs or inactivation system remain to be done, even some are promising [41].

In fact, the take home message would be to target the microenvironment rather than the tumor. Few killing of tumor cells, allowing release of specific TAA, could be sufficient to induce a massive antitumoral immune response when done in combination with reprogrammation of the immunosuppressive inflammatory microenvironment into an antitumoral inflammatory microenvironment. Many believe that combining different approaches will ultimately induce the broadest and most effective immune response to cure HNRB.

Author details

Tala Shekarian[1,2,3,4] and Sandrine Valsesia-Wittmann[1,3,4*]

*Address all correspondence to: sandrine.wittmann@lyon.unicancer.fr

1 Université Lyon 1, Lyon, France

2 INSERM UMR-S1052, CNRS UMR5286, Centre de Recherche en Cancérologie de Lyon, Lyon, France

3 Centre Léon Bérard, Lyon, France

4 PI3 Plateforme d'innovation en immunothérapie, Lyon, France

References

[1] Dunn GP, Bruce AT, Ikeda H, Old LJ, Schreiber RD. Cancer immunoediting: From immunosurveillance to tumor escape. Nature Immunology. 2002 Nov;**3**(11):991-998. DOI: 10.1038/ni1102-991

[2] Dunn GP, Old LJ, Schreiber RD. The immunobiology of cancer immunosurveillance and immunoediting. Immunity. 2004 Aug;**21**(2):137-148. DOI: 10.1016/j.immuni.2004.07.017

[3] Asgharzadeh S, Salo JA, Ji L, Oberthuer A, Fischer M, Berthold F, Hadjidaniel M, Liu CW, Metelitsa LS, Pique-Regi R, Wakamatsu P, Villablanca JG, Kreissman SG, Matthay KK, Shimada H, London WB, Sposto R, Seeger RC. Clinical significance of tumor-associated inflammatory cells in metastatic neuroblastoma. Journal of Clinical Oncology: Official Journal of the American Society of Clinical Oncology. 2012;**30**(28):3525-3532. DOI: 10.1200/JCO.2011.40.9169

[4] Schumacher TN, Schreiber RD. Neoantigens in cancer immunotherapy. Science. 2015: 348;69-74

[5] Pugh TJ, Morozova O, Attiyeh EF, Asgharzadeh S, Wei JS, Auclair D, Carter SL, Cibulskis K, Hanna M, Kiezun A, Kim J, Lawrence MS, Lichenstein L, McKenna A, Pedamallu CS, Ramos AH, Shefler E, Sivachenko A, Sougnez C, Stewart C, Ally A, Birol I, Chiu R, Corbett RD, Hirst M, Jackman SD, Kamoh B, Khodabakshi AH, Krzywinski M, Lo A, Moore RA, Mungall KL, Qian J, Tam A, Thiessen N, Zhao Y, Cole KA, Diamond M, Diskin SJ, Mosse YP, Wood AC, Ji L, Sposto R, Badgett T, London WB, Moyer Y, Gastier-Foster JM, Smith MA, Guidry Auvil JM, Gerhard DS, Hogarty MD, Jones SJ, Lander ES, Gabriel SB, Getz G, Seeger RC, Khan J, Marra MA, Meyerson M, Maris JM. The genetic landscape of high-risk neuroblastoma. Nature Genetics. 2013 Mar;**45**(3):279-284. DOI: 10.1038/ng.2529

[6] Eleveld TF, Oldridge DA, Bernard V, Koster J, Daage LC, Diskin SJ, Schild L, Bentahar NB, Bellini A, Chicard M, Lapouble E, Combaret V, Legoix-Né P, Michon J, Pugh TJ, Hart LS, Rader J, Attiyeh EF, Wei JS, Zhang S, Naranjo A, Gastier-Foster JM, Hogarty MD, Asgharzadeh S, Smith MA, Guidry Auvil JM, Watkins TB, Zwijnenburg DA, Ebus ME, van Sluis P, Hakkert A, van Wezel E, van der Schoot CE, Westerhout EM, Schulte JH, Tytgat GA, Dolman ME, Janoueix-Lerosey I, Gerhard DS, Caron HN, Delattre O, Khan J, Versteeg R, Schleiermacher G, Molenaar JJ, Maris JM. Relapsed neuroblastomas show frequent RAS-MAPK pathway mutations. Nature Genetics. 2015 Aug;**47**(8):864-871. DOI: 10.1038/ng.333

[7] Schramm A, Koster J, Assenov Y, Althoff K, Peifer M, Mahlow E, Odersky A, Beisser D, Ernst C, Henssen AG, et al. Mutational dynamics between primary and relapse neuroblastomas. Nature Genetics. 2015;**47**:872-877

[8] Michot JM, Mazeron R, Dercle L, Ammari S, Canova C, Marabelle A, Rose S, Rubin E, Deutsch E, Soria JC, Ribrag V, Levy A. Abscopal effect in a Hodgkin lymphoma patient treated by an anti-programmed death 1 antibody. European Journal of Cancer. 2016 Oct;**66**:91-94. DOI: 10.1016/j.ejca.2016.06.017

[9] Swart M, Verbrugge I, Beltman JB. Combination approaches with immune-checkpoint blockade in cancer therapy. Frontiers in Oncology. 2016;**6**:233

[10] Yu AL, Gilman AL, Ozkaynak MF, London WB, Kreissman SG, Chen HX, Smith M, Anderson B, Villablanca JG, Matthay KK, Shimada H, Grupp SA, Seeger R, Reynolds CP,

Buxton A, Reisfeld RA, Gillies SD, Cohn SL, Maris JM, Sondel PM; Children's Oncology Group. Anti-GD2 antibody with GM-CSF, interleukin-2, and isotretinoin for neuroblastoma. The New England Journal of Medicine. 2010;**363**(14):1324-1334. DOI: 10.1056/NEJMoa0911123

[11] Dhillon S. Dinutuximab: First global approval. Drugs. 2015;**75**(8):923-927. DOI: 10.1007/s40265-015-0399-5

[12] Yankelevich M, Kondadasula SV, Thakur A, Buck S, Cheung N-KV, Lum LG. Anti-CD3 × anti-GD2 bispecific antibody redirects T-cell cytolytic activity to neuroblastoma targets. Pediatric Blood & Cancer. 2012;**59**(7):1198-1205. DOI: 10.1002/pbc.24237

[13] Cordeau M, Belounis A, Lelaidier M, Cordeiro P, Sartelet H, Herblot S, Duval M. Efficient killing of high risk neuroblastoma using natural killer cells activated by plasmacytoid dendritic cells. PLoS ONE. 2016;**11**(10):e0164401. DOI: 10.1371/journal.pone.0164401

[14] Semeraro M, Rusakiewicz S, Minard-Colin V, Delahaye NF, Enot D, Vély F, Marabelle A, Papoular B, Piperoglou C, Ponzoni M, Perri P, Tchirkov A, Matta J, Lapierre V, Shekarian T, Valsesia-Wittmann S, Commo F, Prada N, Poirier-Colame V, Bressac B, Cotteret S, Brugieres L, Farace F, Chaput N, Kroemer G, Valteau-Couanet D, Zitvogel L. Zitvogel L. Clinical impact of the NKp30/B7-H6 axis in high-risk neuroblastoma patients. Science Translational Medicine. 2015;**7**(283):283ra55. DOI: 10.1126/scitranslmed.aaa2327

[15] Lee DW, Kochenderfer JN, Stetler-Stevenson M, Cui YK, Delbrook C, Feldman SA, Fry TJ, Orentas R, Sabatino M, Shah NN, et al. T cells expressing CD19 chimeric antigen receptors for acute lymphoblastic leukaemia in children and young adults: A phase 1 dose-escalation trial. Lancet. 2015;385:517-528

[16] Long AH, Haso WM, Shern JF, Wanhainen KM, Murgai M, Ingaramo M, Smith JP, Walker AJ, Kohler ME, Venkateshwara VR, et al. 4-1BB costimulation ameliorates T cell exhaustion induced by tonic signaling of chimeric antigen receptors. Nature Medicine. 2015;**21**:581-590

[17] Pule MA, Savoldo B, Myers GD, Rossig C, Russell HV, Dotti G, Huls MH, Liu E, Gee AP, Mei Z, et al. Virus-specific T cells engineered to coexpress tumor-specific receptors: Persistence and antitumor activity in individuals with neuroblastoma. Nature Medicine. 2008;**14**:1264-1270

[18] Heczey A, Louis CU, Savoldo B, Dakhova O, Grilley BJ, Gee A, Dotti GP, Heslop HE, Rooney CM, Brenner MK. Autologous T cells expressing a GD2 specific chimeric antigen receptor with CD28 and OX40 costimulatory endodomains for children with neuroblastoma. Paper presented at: Advances in Neuroblastoma Research Congress. 2016

[19] Gonzalez S, Naranjo A, Serrano LM, Chang W-C, Wright CL, Jensen MC. Genetic engineering of cytolytic T lymphocytes for adoptive T-cell therapy of neuroblastoma. The Journal of Gene Medicine. 2004;**6**(6):704-711. DOI: 10.1002/jgm.489

[20] Künkele A, Taraseviciute A, Finn LS, Johnson AJ, Berger C, Finney O, Chang A, Rolczynski LS, Brown C, Mgebroff S, Berger M, Park JR, Jensen MC. Preclinical Assessment of CD171-Directed CAR T-cell Adoptive Therapy for Childhood Neuroblastoma: CE7

Epitope Target Safety and Product Manufacturing Feasibility. Clin Cancer Res. 2017 Jan 15;**23**(2):466-477. doi: 10.1158/1078-0432.CCR-16-0354. Epub 2016 Jul 7.

[21] Singh N, Kulikovskaya I, Barrett DM, Binder-Scholl G, Jakobsen B, Martinez D, Pawel B, June CH, Kalos MD, Grupp SA. T cells targeting NY-ESO-1 demonstrate efficacy against disseminated neuroblastoma. OncoImmunology. 2016;**5**(1):e1040216. DOI: 10.1080/2162402X.2015.1040216

[22] Chitu V, Stanley ER. Colony-stimulating factor-1 in immunity and inflammation. Current Opinion in Immunology. 2006;**18**(1):39-48. DOI: 10.1016/j.coi.2005.11.006

[23] Strachan DC, Ruffell B, Oei Y, Bissell MJ, Coussens LM, Pryer N, Daniel D. CSF1R inhibition delays cervical and mammary tumor growth in murine models by attenuating the turnover of tumor-associated macrophages and enhancing infiltration by CD8 + T cells. OncoImmunology. 2013;**2**(12):e26968. DOI: 10.4161/onci.26968

[24] Mao Y, Eissler N, Blanc KL, Johnsen JI, Kogner P, Kiessling R. Targeting suppressive myeloid cells potentiates checkpoint inhibitors to control spontaneous neuroblastoma. Clinical Cancer Research. 2016;**22**(15):3849-59. DOI: 10.1158/1078-0432.CCR-15-1912. Epub 2016 Mar 8.

[25] Cappel C, Huenecke S, Suemmerer A, Erben S, Rettinger E, Pfirrmann V, Heinze A, Zimmermann O, Klingebiel T, Ullrich E, Bader P, Bremm M. Cytotoxic potential of IL-15-activated cytokine-induced killer cells against human neuroblastoma cells. Pediatric Blood & Cancer. 2016;**63**(12):2230-2239. DOI: 10.1002/pbc.26147

[26] Russell SJ, Peng K-W, Bell JC. Oncolytic virotherapy. Nature Biotechnology. 2012; **30**(7):658-670. DOI: 10.1038/nbt.2287

[27] You Z, Fischer DC, Tong X, Hasenburg A, Aguilar-Cordova E, Kieback DG. Coxsackievirus–adenovirus receptor expression in ovarian cancer cell lines is associated with increased adenovirus transduction efficiency and transgene expression. Cancer Gene Therapy. 2001;**8**(3):168-175. DOI: 10.1038/sj.cgt.7700284

[28] Hammond AL, Plemper RK, Zhang J, Schneider U, Russell SJ, Cattaneo R. Single-chain antibody displayed on a recombinant measles virus confers entry through the tumor-associated carcinoembryonic antigen. Journal of Virology. 2001;**75**(5):2087-2096. DOI: 10.1128/JVI.75.5.2087-2096.2001

[29] Bischoff JR, Kirn DH, Williams A, Heise C, Horn S, Muna M, Ng L, Nye JA, Sampson-Johannes A, Fattaey A, McCormick F. An adenovirus mutant that replicates selectively in p53-deficient human tumor cells. Science (New York, N.Y.). 1996;274(5286):373-6. http://www.ncbi.nlm.nih.gov/pubmed/8832876

[30] Lin E, Nemunaitis J. Oncolytic viral therapies. Cancer Gene Therapy. 2004;**11**(10):643-664. DOI: 10.1038/sj.cgt.7700733

[31] Fukuhara H, Ino Y, Todo T. Oncolytic virus therapy: A new era of cancer treatment at dawn. Cancer Science. 2016;**107**(10):1373-1379. DOI: 10.1111/cas.13027

[32] Kaufman HL, Kohlhapp FJ, Zloza A. Oncolytic viruses: A new class of immunotherapy drugs. Nature Reviews Drug Discovery. 2015;**14**(9):642-662. DOI: 10.1038/nrd4663

[33] Valsesia-Wittmann S, Magdeleine M, Dupasquier S, Garin E, Jallas AC, Combaret V, Krause A, Leissner P, Puisieux A. Oncogenic cooperation between H-Twist and N-Myc overrides failsafe programs in cancer cells. Cancer Cell. 2004;**6**(6):625-630. DOI: 10.1016/j.ccr.2004.09.033

[34] Selmi A, de Saint-Jean M, Jallas AC, Garin E, Hogarty MD, Bénard J, Puisieux A, Marabelle A, Valsesia-Wittmann S. TWIST1 is a direct transcriptional target of MYCN and MYC in neuroblastoma. Cancer Letters. 2015 Feb 1;**357**(1):412-418. DOI: 10.1016/j.canlet.2014.11.056

[35] Lutz W, Fulda S, Jeremias I, Debatin KM, Schwab M. MycN and IFNgamma cooperate in apoptosis of human neuroblastoma cells. Oncogene. 1998;**17**(3):339-346. DOI: 10.1038/sj.onc.1200201

[36] Edsjö A, Nilsson H, Vandesompele J, Karlsson J, Pattyn F, Culp LA, Speleman F, Påhlman S. Neuroblastoma cells with overexpressed MYCN retain their capacity to undergo neuronal differentiation. Laboratory Investigation; A Journal of Technical Methods and Pathology. 2004;**84**(4):406-417. DOI: 10.1038/labinvest.3700061

[37] Breit S, Schwab M. Suppression of MYC by high expression of NMYC in human neuroblastoma cells. Journal of Neuroscience Research. 1989;**24**(1):21-28. DOI: 10.1002/jnr.490240105

[38] Westermann F, Muth D, Benner A, Bauer T, Henrich KO, Oberthuer A, Brors B, Beissbarth T, Vandesompele J, Pattyn F, Hero B, König R, Fischer M, Schwab M. Distinct transcriptional MYCN/c-MYC activities are associated with spontaneous regression or malignant progression in neuroblastomas. Genome Biology. 2008;**9**(10):R150. DOI: 10.1186/gb-2008-9-10-r150

[39] Qin Q, Xu Y, He T, Qin C, Xu J. Normal and disease-related biological functions of Twist1 and underlying molecular mechanisms. Cell Research. 2012 Jan;**22**(1):90-106. DOI: 10.1038/cr.2011.144

[40] Naujokat C, Steinhart R. Salinomycin as a drug for targeting human cancer stem cells. Journal of Biomedicine and Biotechnology. 2012;**2012**:950658. DOI: 10.1155/2012/950658. Epub 2012 Nov 21.

[41] Dewangan J, Srivastava S, Rath SK. Salinomycin: A new paradigm in cancer therapy. Tumour Biology. 2017 Mar;**39**(3):1010428317695035. doi: 10.1177/1010428317695035

[42] Low-Marchelli JM, Ardi VC, Vizcarra EA, van Rooijen N, Quigley JP, Yang J. Twist1 induces CCL2 and recruits macrophages to promote angiogenesis. Cancer Research. 2013 Jan 15;**73**(2):662-671. DOI: 10.1158/0008-5472.CAN-12-0653

[43] Mironchik Y, Winnard PT Jr, Vesuna F, Kato Y, Wildes F, Pathak AP, Kominsky S, Artemov D, Bhujwalla Z, Van Diest P, Burger H, Glackin C, Raman V. Twist overexpression induces in vivo angiogenesis and correlates with chromosomal instability in breast cancer. Cancer Research. 2005 Dec 1;**65**(23):10801-10809

[44] Ginhoux F, Jung S. Monocytes and macrophages: Developmental pathways and tissue homeostasis. Nature Reviews Immunology. 2014 Jun;**14**(6):392-404. DOI: 10.1038/nri3671

[45] Mosser DM, Edwards JP. Exploring the full spectrum of macrophage activation. Nature Reviews Immunology. 2008 Dec;**8**(12):958-969. DOI: 10.1038/nri2448

[46] Murray PJ, Wynn TA. Protective and pathogenic functions of macrophage subsets. Nature Reviews Immunology. 2011 Oct 14;**11**(11):723-737. DOI: 10.1038/nri3073

[47] Wang X, Chang X, Zhuo G, Sun M, Yin K. Twist and miR-34a are involved in the generation of tumor-educated myeloid-derived suppressor cells. International Journal of Molecular Sciences. 2013 Oct 14;**14**(10):20459-20477. DOI: 10.3390/ijms141020459

[48] Yamaguchi H, Maruyama T, Urade Y, Nagata S. Immunosuppression via adenosine receptor activation by adenosine monophosphate released from apoptotic cells. Elife. 2014 Mar 25;**3**:e02172. DOI: 10.7554/eLife.02172

[49] Pello OM, Chèvre R, Laoui D, De Juan A, Lolo F, Andrés-Manzano MJ, Serrano M, Van Ginderachter JA, Andrés V. In vivo inhibition of c-myc in myeloid cells impairs tumor-associated macrophage maturation and pro-tumoral activities. PLoS One. 2012;**7**(9):e45399. DOI: 10.1371/journal.pone.0045399

[50] Chiocca EA, Rabkin SD. Oncolytic viruses and their application to cancer immunotherapy. Cancer Immunology Research. 2014;**2**(4):295-300. DOI: 10.1158/2326-6066.CIR-14-0015